Obstetrics, Gynaecology and Women's Health
on the move

Obstetrics, Gynaecology and Women's Health
on the move

Authors: **Amie Clifford, Claire Kelly, Christopher Yau**
Contributing author: Sally Hallam
Editorial Advisor: **Stephen C. Smith**
Series Editors: **Rory Mackinnon, Sally Keat, Thomas Locke and Andrew Walker**

**HODDER
ARNOLD**
AN HACHETTE UK COMPANY

First published in Great Britain in 2012 by
Hodder Arnold, an imprint of Hodder Education, a division of Hachette UK
338 Euston Road, London NW1 3BH

http://www.hodderarnold.com

Whilst the advice and information in this book are believed to be true and accurate at the
date of going to press, neither the author[s] nor the publisher can accept any legal
responsibility or liability for any errors or omissions that may be made. In particular, (but
without limiting the generality of the preceding disclaimer) every effort has been made to
check drug dosages; however, it is still possible that errors have been missed. Furthermore,
dosage schedules are constantly being revised and new side-effects recognized. For these
reasons the reader is strongly urged to consult the drug companies' printed instructions,
and their websites, before administering any of the drugs recommended in this book.

British Library Cataloguing in Publication Data
A catalogue record for this book is available from the British Library

Library of Congress Cataloging-in-Publication Data
A catalog record for this book is available from the Library of Congress

ISBN-13   978-1-444-14563-2

1 2 3 4 5 6 7 8 9 10
Commissioning Editor: Joanna Koster
Project Editor: Stephen Clausard
Production Controller: Francesca Wardell
Cover Design: Amina Dudhia

Cover image © Sebastian Kaulitzki – Fotolia &© franckreporter/istockphoto.com
(smartphone)

Typeset in 10/12pt Adobe Garamond Pro Regular by Datapage (India) Pvt. Ltd.
Printed and bound in India

What do you think about this book? Or any other Hodder Arnold title?
Please visit our website: www.hodderarnold.com

Contents

Preface

Obstetrics and Gynaecology is a challenging specialty encompassing aspects of both medicine and surgery. It requires a considerable knowledge base, and presents a unique array of problems, which can prove daunting for both medical students and junior doctors alike.

Our challenge with this book was to try to present these fascinating but difficult subjects in an informative, yet accessible way. We have therefore tried to keep the text as concise as possible, and included many flow diagrams and summary tables. We hope that this approach will help you connect with the topics and make them easier to understand.

Unlike many books dealing with Obstetrics and Gynaecology, we have also included a chapter on breast diseases. As such, we hope that this book will offer you a comprehensive overview of women's health as a whole.

Whether you are a medical student studying women's health, or a junior doctor working in Obstetrics and Gynaecology, we hope this book will support you in your study and your work.

Finally, we would welcome any feedback or suggestions for improvements you may have. Please feel free to contact us.

AUTHORS

Amie Clifford MBChB – Foundation Year 2 doctor, Northern General Hospital, Sheffield, UK
Claire Kelly BMedSci – Fifth Year student doctor, University of Sheffield, Sheffield, UK
Christopher Yau MBChB – Foundation Year 1 doctor, Musgrove Park Hospital, Taunton, UK

CONTRIBUTING AUTHOR

Sally Hallam BMedSci MBChB – Foundation Year 2 doctor, Chelsea and Westminster Hospital, London, UK

EDITORIAL ADVISOR

Stephen C. Smith BSc MBChB FRCOG MFFP DM – Consultant in Obstetrics and Gynaecology, Chesterfield Royal Hospital NHS Foundation Trust, Chesterfield, UK; Operating Surgeon and Abortion Practitioner, BPAS, UK

EDITOR-IN-CHIEF

Rory Mackinnon BSc MBChB – Foundation Year 2 doctor, Northern
General Hospital, Sheffield, UK

SERIES EDITORS

Sally Keat BMedSci MBChB – Foundation Year 1 doctor, Northern
General Hospital, Sheffield, UK
Thomas Locke BSc MBChB – Foundation Year 1 doctor, Northern
General Hospital, Sheffield, UK
Andrew Walker BMedSci MBChB – Specialist Trainee Year 1 doctor in
Medicine, Chesterfield Royal Hospital, Chesterfield, Derbyshire, UK

Acknowledgements

We are very grateful to: Mr Stephen Smith for his continuing advice, support and patience as editorial adviser; Ms Lynda Wyld for the expertise she has offered in relation to diseases of the breast; and Mr Tony Hollingworth for undertaking the invaluable role of reviewing the final manuscript.

We would also like to thank all the staff at the Clinical Skills Centre, Northern General Hospital, Sheffield, for allowing us to use their facilities.

Finally we would like to extend our heartfelt thanks to all our families and friends for the support they have given during the writing of this book.

The following figures have been reproduced from Baker P and Kenny L. *Obstetrics by Ten Teachers. 9th edition.* London: Hodder Arnold, 2011, with kind permission from the authors: 1.3, 1.4, 5.1, 6.1, 6.2, 6.4, 6.5, 6.9, 7.1, 7.3, 7.4, 8.1

The following figures have been reproduced Monga A. and Dobbs S. *Gynaecology by Ten Teachers. 19th edition.* London: Hodder Arnold, 2011, with kind permission from the authors: 10.7, 10.8, 13.1, 18.1, 18.2, 18.3, 18.4, 18.5, 19.2, 19.3, 19.4, 21.1, 23.1

List of abbreviations

- AED: anti-epileptic drug
- AIDS: acquired immunodeficiency syndrome
- APH: antepartum haemorrhage
- ARM: artificial rupture of membranes
- b.p.m.: beats per minute
- BMI: body mass index
- BP: blood pressure
- BSO: bilateral salpingo-oophorectomy
- BV: bacterial vaginosis
- CIN: cervical intra-epithelial neoplasia
- CMV: cytomegalovirus
- CNS: central nervous system
- COCP: combined oral contraceptive pill
- COPD: chronic obstructive pulmonary disease
- CSF: cerebrospinal fluid
- CT: computed tomography
- CTG: cardiotocography
- CVS: chorionic villus sampling
- D&E: dilation and evacuation
- DCDA: dichorionic, diamniotic
- DIC: disseminated intravascular coagulation
- DUB: dysfunctional uterine bleeding
- DVT: deep vein thrombosis
- ECV: external cephalic version
- EDD: estimated date of delivery
- EGFR2: epidermal growth factor receptor 2
- ER: oestrogen receptor
- FBC: full blood count
- FHR: fetal heart rate
- FSH: follicle-stimulating hormone
- FT_3/FT_4: free thyroid hormones
- GBS: group B *Streptococcus*
- GFR: glomerular filtration rate
- GnRH: gonadotrophin-releasing hormone
- GSI: genuine stress incontinence
- GTD: gestational trophoblastic disease
- GTN: gestational trophoblastic neoplasia
- Hb: haemoglobin
- HbA_{1c}: haemoglobin A_{1c}

- hCG: human chorionic gonadotrophin
- HELLP: haemolysis, elevated liver enzymes and low platelets
- HER2: human epidermal growth factor receptor 2
- HIV: human immunodeficiency virus
- HMB: heavy menstrual bleeding
- HPO: hypothalamic–pituitary–ovarian
- HPV: human papillomavirus
- HRT: hormone replacement therapy
- HSG: hysterosalpingogram
- HSV: herpes simplex virus
- IBS: irritable bowel syndrome
- IM: intramuscularly
- IMB: inter-menstrual bleeding
- iu: international units
- IUCD: intra-uterine coil device
- IUGR: intra-uterine growth restriction
- IUS: intra-uterine system
- IVF: *in vitro* fertilization
- LFT: liver function test
- LH: luteinizing hormone
- LMP: last menstrual period
- LSCS: lower segment caesarean section
- MCDA: monochorionic, diamniotic
- MCMA: monochorionic, monoamniotic
- MDT: multidisciplinary team
- MMR: measles, mumps and rubella vaccine
- MRI: magnetic resonance imaging
- NICE: National Institute for Health and Clinical Excellence
- NSAID: non-steroidal anti-inflammatory drug
- NT: nuchal translucency
- OA: occiput anterior
- OP: occiput posterior
- OT: occiput transverse
- PCOS: polycystic ovary syndrome
- PE: pulmonary embolus
- PID: pelvic inflammatory disease
- PMS: pre-menstrual syndrome
- POP: progesterone-only pill
- PPH: postpartum haemorrhage
- PPROM: pre-term/pre-labour rupture of membranes
- PRN: *pro re nata*
- PV: per vaginum
- RMI: risk malignancy index

- SFH: symphysis–fundal height
- SHBG: steroid hormone-binding globulin
- SROM: spontaneous rupture of membranes
- STI: sexually transmitted infection
- SUI: stress urinary incontinence
- T_4: thyroxine
- TAH: total abdominal hysterectomy
- TENS: transcutaneous electrical nerve stimulation
- TNM: tumour–node–metastasis staging system
- TSH: thyroid-stimulating hormone
- TTTS: twin-to-twin transfusion syndrome
- TVS: transvaginal ultrasound scan
- TVT: tension-free vaginal tape
- TVT-O: transobturator tape
- USS: ultrasound scan
- UTI: urinary tract infection
- VIN: vulval intra-epithelial neoplasia
- VTE: venous thromboembolic disease

An explanation of the text

The book is divided into four parts: obstetrics, gynaecology, women's health and a self-assessment section. We have used bullet-points to keep the text concise and brief and supplemented this with a range of diagrams, pictures and MICRO-boxes (explained below).

> ## MICRO-facts
> These boxes expand on the text and contain clinically relevant facts and memorable summaries of the essential information.

> ### MICRO-print
> These boxes contain additional information to the text that may interest certain readers but is not essential for everybody to learn.

> ### MICRO-case
> These boxes contain clinical cases relevant to the text and include a number of summary bullet points to highlight the key learning objectives.

> ### MICRO-reference
> These boxes contain references to important clinical research and national guidance.

Normal range values are given for most tests in this book as a guideline for your knowledge. Please note that ranges differ between laboratories and therefore you should always use figures from your own institution to interpret results.

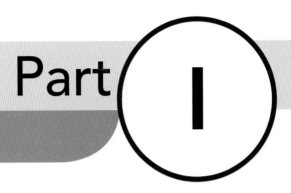

Part I

Obstetrics

Obstetrics: history and examination

1.1 GENERAL PRINCIPLES

DEFINITIONS

- Gravidity:
    - This is the total number of pregnancies.
    - This includes the current pregnancy and any miscarriages, ectopic pregnancies or terminations.
    - A **primigravida** is a woman in her first pregnancy.
    - A **nulligravida** has never been pregnant.
    - A **multigravida** has been pregnant more than once.
- Parity:
    - This is expressed as $X + Y$, where X is the number of deliveries after 24 weeks, whether alive or stillbirth, and Y is the total number of miscarriages, ectopic pregnancies and terminations.
    - A **nulliparous** woman has not delivered a baby (beyond 24 weeks' gestation).
    - A **primiparous** woman has delivered a baby once (beyond 24 weeks' gestation).
    - A **multiparous** woman has delivered more than one baby (beyond 24 weeks' gestation).

MICRO-facts

In practice, although they are not equivalent terms, **'primiparous'** or **'primip'** is often used interchangeably with 'primagravida' to refer to a woman in her first pregnancy.

- A twin pregnancy counts as a single pregnancy for gravidity but gives a parity of two.

> ## MICRO-facts
>
> Jane is pregnant. She has two children, which she delivered at term, and previously had one miscarriage at 14 weeks.
>
> - She is **gravida** 4, **para** 2 + 1, or G4 P2 + 1.
>
> Mary is pregnant with twins. She has had two previous miscarriages, one at 10 weeks and another at 12 weeks.
>
> - She is **gravida** 3, **para** 0 + 2, or G3 P0 + 2.

1.2 OBSTETRIC HISTORY

PERSONAL DETAILS

- Age.
- Gestation: how many weeks?
- Gravidity and parity.

PRESENTING COMPLAINT

- For example, abdominal pain, bleeding, nausea and vomiting.

CURRENT PREGNANCY

- Last menstrual period (LMP) and estimated date of delivery (EDD).
- Planned or unplanned?
- Spontaneous or assisted pregnancy (e.g. *in vitro* fertilization)?
- Menstrual history, including cycle length.
- Contraceptive history.
- Antenatal history:
    - complications;
    - attendance at antenatal appointments;
    - abnormal test/scan results;
    - midwife/consultant-led care.

> ## MICRO-facts
>
> **Naegele's rule**
>
> For a woman with a 28 day menstrual cycle, the estimated date of delivery (EDD) is calculated by:
>
> (Last menstrual period (LMP) − 3 months) + 7 days + 1 year
>
> To correct for cycles longer or shorter than 28 days, **add** or **subtract** the difference from 28 days to the EDD, e.g.
>
> LMP = 1/1/2011 in a woman with 30 day cycles; EDD = 10/10/2011
>
> Obstetric 'wheels' are also used to quickly calculate the EDD.

PAST OBSTETRIC HISTORY

- For each pregnancy:
    - When did it occur (year)?
    - Did it result in a live birth?
    - What was the gestation (i.e. the length of that pregnancy)?
    - What was the mode of delivery, e.g. vaginal, caesarean section, etc.?
    - What was the birthweight and sex of the baby?
    - Were there any antenatal, intra-partum or post-natal maternal and fetal complications?
    - Does the child have any health problems?
- History of terminations/miscarriages/ectopic pregnancies:
    - At what gestation did it occur?
    - What was the management and were there any complications?
    - What was the indication for any terminations?
- Rhesus status and anti-D vaccinations.

MICRO-facts

A personal and family history of the following should be recorded:
- heart disease;
- hypertension and pre-eclampsia;
- diabetes;
- renal disease;
- jaundice;
- epilepsy;
- venous thromboembolic disease;
- thrombophilia;
- psychiatric disorders.

PAST GYNAECOLOGICAL HISTORY

See 10.1 History in Chapter 10, Gynaecology: history and examination.

CERVICAL SMEAR HISTORY

- Up-to-date with screening? Date of last smear.
- History of abnormal smears, including their investigation and management.

PAST MEDICAL AND SURGICAL HISTORY

- Operations.

DRUG HISTORY

- Current medications.

Obstetrics

- Recreational drug use.
- Did the patient take folic acid supplementation?

ALLERGIES

- To anything, e.g. drug, foodstuff or latex.
- Elicit exactly what the reaction was.

FAMILY HISTORY

- Congenital abnormalities.

SOCIAL HISTORY

- Who does the woman live with?
- Type of accommodation.
- Does she have a supportive partner? If not, who will give her support?
- Occupation.
- Smoking and alcohol history.

1.3 EXAMINATIONS

GENERAL EXAMINATION

- General appearance.
- Measure weight and height; calculate body mass index.
- Blood pressure.
- Oedema: facial, sacral, palmar or pedal.
- Signs of anaemia.
- Dipstick the urine for glycosuria and proteinuria.

MEDICAL EXAMINATION

- If clinically indicated, e.g. optic fundi in a hypertensive patient.

OBSTETRIC EXAMINATION

> **MICRO-facts**
>
> Positioning for the obstetric examination:
> - semi-recumbent;
> - exposed from the lower chest to below the hips;
> - cover the woman's lap with a sheet.

- **Inspection**:
  - Abdominal distension:
    - Size and symmetry.

- Linea nigra:
  - A dark line of hyperpigmented skin visible in the midline of the abdomen from the umbilicus to the pubis.
  - It is common during pregnancy.
- Striae gravidarum or 'stretch marks' are also common.
- Scars:
  - For example, caesarean section (lower segment or vertical incision), laparotomy, laparoscopy.
- Umbilicus:
  - Is it everted? This may suggest polyhydramnios or multiple gestation.
- Fetal movements (may be seen after 24 weeks).
- **Palpation**:
  - The uterus may be palpable abdominally at 12–14 weeks:
    - The height of the fundus increases with gestation (see Fig. 1.1).
  - To measure the symphysis–fundal height (SFH):
    - Feel for the fundus as shown in Fig. 1.2a using the ulnar side of your hand.
    - Palpate the upper border of the symphysis pubis.
    - Measure from the symphysis pubis to the top of the fundus using a tape measure with the markings face down. Turn over the tape. Record the measurement on a SFH chart (in centimetres).

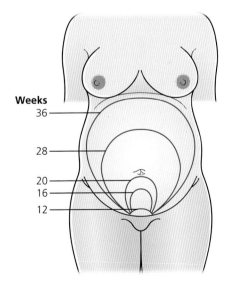

Fig. 1.1 Palpating the size of the uterus can be used to estimate gestation.

(a) Palpate the fundus

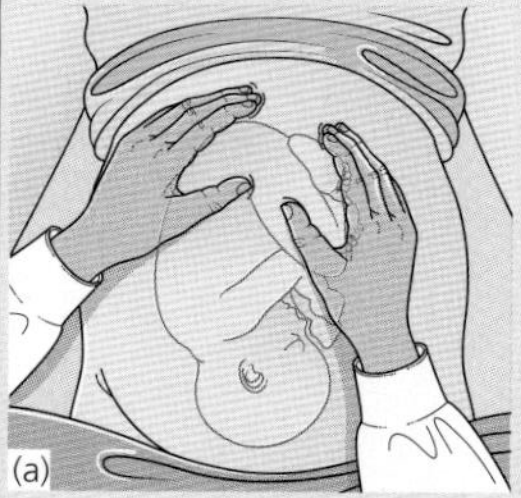

- Face the woman's head
- Use the ulnar border of your hand to palpate the fundus
- Determine which fetal part is at the fundus: usually the head or buttocks (breech)
- A head is hard and ballotable
- A breech is softer and cannot be balloted

(b) Examine the fetal parts

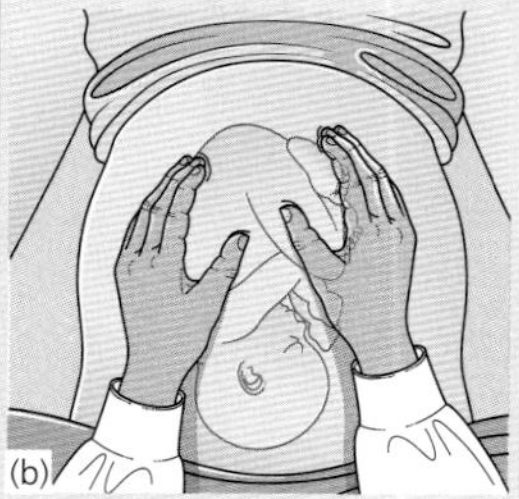

- Face the woman's head
- With the flat of one hand, apply pressure to one side of the uterus
- On the opposite side use the flats of your fingers to palpate the fetal parts. Perform for both sides
- Can you feel more than one head and one breech? Suspect multiple gestation
- Confirm the lie and determine which side the fetal back is
- Judge the liquor volume
- Feel for fetal movements

(c) Determine the presentation

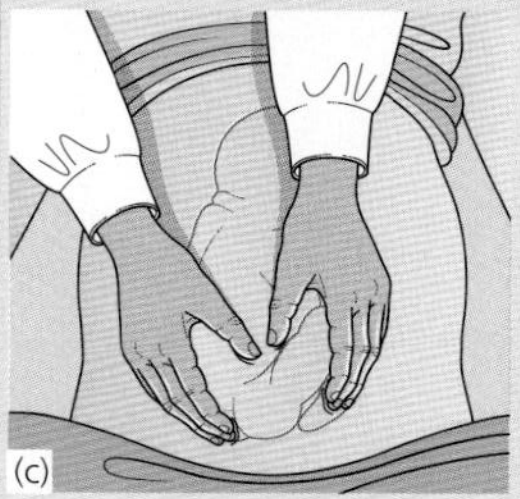

- Face the woman's feet
- Use both hands to palpate above the symphysis pubis
- Determine which part of the fetus is lowest: usually the head or breech.

(d) Determine whether the presenting part is engaged

- Palpate as shown in part (c) to determine if the presenting part is mobile
- If it is mobile, it is not engaged
- For a cephalic presentation, use the fingers of your hand to estimate how many fifths of the head you can feel abdominally
- If two finger breadths or less is palpable, the head is engaged

Fig. 1.2 (a–d) Palpating the fetal parts.

MICRO-facts

After 24 weeks' gestation the symphysis–fundal height (SFH) (in cm) should equal the gestation (in weeks) $\pm 2\,cm$. If the SFH is larger than expected, it is known as 'large for dates' and may be due to:

- macrosomia;
- multiple gestation;
- polyhydramnios.

A smaller SFH than expected is called 'small for dates'. This may be due to:

- intra-uterine growth restriction;
- oligohydramnios.

- Palpating the fetal parts. Use the four steps shown in Fig. 1.2 to determine the:
  - lie;
  - liquor volume;
  - presentation;
  - engagement.
- **Lie**:
  - The relationship of the longitudinal axis of the fetus (i.e. its spine) to the longitudinal axis of the uterus.

Table 1.1 Types of lie.

LIE	DEFINITION	PRESENTATION
Longitudinal (see Fig. 1.3a)	Fetal spine is parallel to long axis of the uterus	Cephalic or breech
Transverse (see Fig. 1.3b)	Fetal spine is at 90° to the long axis of the uterus	Presenting part will be the arm/shoulder/trunk
Oblique (see Fig. 1.3c)	Fetus lies diagonally across the uterus	This is unstable, and may revert to longitudinal or transverse lie

- **Liquor volume**:
  - This is judged by how easily the fetal parts are palpated.
  - Oligohydramnios: there is little liquor; therefore, the fetal parts may be easier to palpate.
  - Polyhydramnios: there is excess liquor; it may be difficult to palpate the fetal parts. Depending on the severity of polyhydramnios, the fetus may be ballotable. Fig. 1.3

Obstetrics

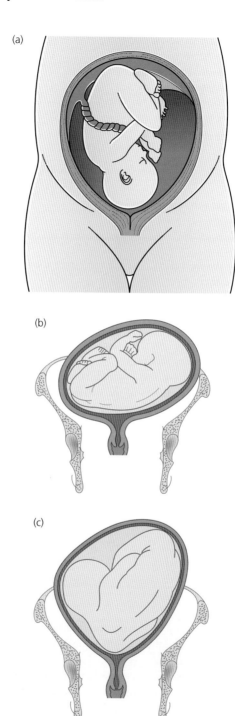

(a)

(b)

(c)

Fig. 1.3 (a) Longitudinal, (b) transverse and (c) oblique lie.

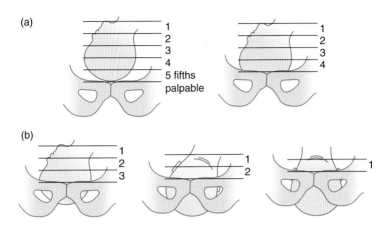

Fig. 1.4 Palpation of the fetal head to assess engagement.

- **Presentation**:
  - The part of the fetus that occupies the lower part of the uterus or the pelvis.
  - Since the lie is most commonly longitudinal, this is usually **cephalic** (head) or **breech** (buttocks).
- **Engagement (see Fig. 1.4)**:
  - This is a measure of how far the fetus has descended into the pelvis.
  - Usually it is only used for cephalic presentations.
  - The fetus is 'engaged' when the widest diameter of the presenting part is through the pelvic brim.
  - Since the size of the fetal head is roughly the same as the examiner's hand, fingers can be used to estimate the fifths of the head palpable.
  - The head is engaged when two finger breadths or less is palpable abdominally.
  - In a primigravida this usually occurs by 37 weeks. In multiparous women it may not occur until the onset of labour.

- **Auscultation**:
  - Listen over the fetal anterior shoulder (between the fetal head and the mother's umbilicus) with a hand-held Doppler device.

MICRO-facts

A normal fetal heart rate is **110–160** b.p.m. and **regular**.

Obstetrics

2

Antenatal care

2.1 INTRODUCTION

AIMS OF ANTENATAL CARE

- To improve maternal and fetal health and prevent disease.
- To screen for and manage fetal and maternal disease.
- To educate and support the pregnant woman and her family.
- To plan for labour.

MIDWIFE AND GP VS. OBSTETRICIAN-LED CARE

- Midwives and GPs can manage uncomplicated pregnancies.
- Common indications for obstetrician-led care include:
  - Medical:
    - hypertensive disease;
    - diabetes (insulin dependent).
  - Older women (over 40 years).
  - Previous caesarean section.
  - Previous complicated pregnancy.
- A full list can be found in the National Institute for Health and Clinical Excellence guidelines.

> **MICRO-reference**
> National Institute for Health and Clinical Excellence. Antenatal care: routine care for the healthy pregnant woman. NICE Clinical Guidance 62. London, UK: NICE, 2008. Available at http://guidance.nice.org.uk/CG62

2.2 ADVICE IN PREGNANCY

GENERAL ADVICE

- Work:
  - Assess potential occupational risk factors, e.g. exposure to radiation.

- Supplementation:
  - Advise daily folic acid (400 μg): pre-conception to 12 weeks' gestation.
  - Identify women at high risk of vitamin D deficiency.
  - Avoid vitamin A supplements:
    - high intake during early pregnancy is teratogenic.

MICRO-facts

Folic acid reduces the risk of neural tube defects, e.g. spina bifida.

- Food:
  - Avoid liver (high vitamin A).
  - To reduce the risk of listeriosis, avoid:
    - unpasteurized milk and soft cheese;
    - undercooked food;
    - pâté.
  - To reduce the risk of *Salmonella*, avoid:
    - raw or partially cooked eggs and meat.
- Alcohol:
  - **Pre-conception to 3 months**:
    - avoid alcohol completely owing to the increased risk of miscarriage.
  - **3 months to term**:
    - the maximum safe limit is one or two units once or twice a week.
  - Avoid binge-drinking (>7.5 units at one time).
- Prescribed and over-the-counter drugs:
  - Women should be advised to seek advice from a pharmacist before taking medicines.
- Give smoking cessation advice.
- Exercise:
  - Encourage moderate exercise, including specific pelvic floor exercises.
  - Advise the woman to avoid high-impact or contact sports and scuba diving.
- Travel:
  - Pregnant women should wear a seatbelt 'above and below the bump, not over it'.
  - The safety of flying changes throughout pregnancy: pregnant women should discuss any air travel with their midwife.
  - Women should organize adequate health insurance and carry their pregnancy notes with them.

Obstetrics

PRE-LABOUR COUNSELLING

- Women are encouraged to write a birth plan:
    - This includes decisions about the place of birth, pain control and interventions if the labour is complicated.
- Location:
    - The woman may choose where to deliver:
        - at home;
        - in a community unit (midwife-led unit);
        - in hospital (midwife-led unit or consultant-led unit).
    - Women with complicated pregnancies are likely to be managed in a consultant-led unit.

MICRO-reference

An example of a birth plan: http://www.nhs.uk/planners/pregnancycar-eplanner/pages/BirthPlan.aspx

---

2.3 THE ANTENATAL SCREENING PROGRAMME

SCHEDULE OF APPOINTMENTS

- For ideal antenatal care, the woman would present to her GP pre-conceptually.
- For an uncomplicated pregnancy:
    - Parous women have eight appointments.
    - Nulliparous women have 11 appointments:
        - this allows closer monitoring of blood pressure (BP), symphysis–fundal height and proteinuria.
    - There is an appointment at 41 weeks for women who have not yet delivered.
    - Fig. 2.1 gives an overview of these appointments.

THE BOOKING VISIT

- This should take place by 10 weeks (this is the national target).
- A full obstetric history is taken to identify high-risk pregnancies.
- **Screening tests**:
    - BP.
    - Body mass index.
    - Urine:
        - Proteinuria.
        - Bacteriuria.

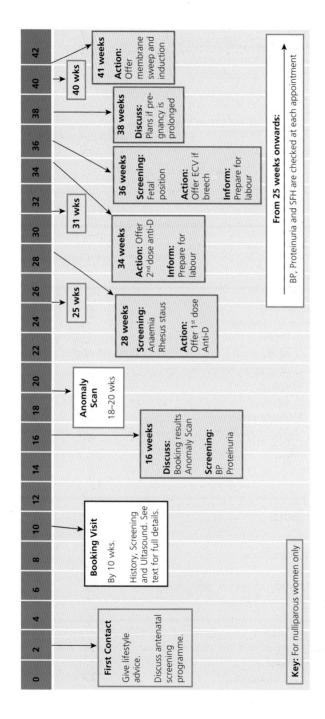

Fig. 2.1 Schedule of antenatal appointments.

- **Blood tests:**
  - Full blood count: anaemia.
  - Blood group and rhesus D status.
  - Red cell alloantibodies.
  - Haemoglobinopathies: in at-risk women.
  - Glucose.
  - Blood tests for Down's syndrome.
  - Infection:
    - ○ hepatitis B;
    - ○ human immunodeficiency virus;
    - ○ rubella;
    - ○ syphilis.

MICRO-print

It is very important to properly counsel and consent women for each screening test.

- **Ultrasound:**
  - Gestational age:
    - ○ between 10 and 14 weeks the crown–rump length (from the top of the head to the bottom of the buttocks) is used to confirm/determine gestational age.
  - Viability:
    - ○ whether the fetal heart beat can be identified.
  - Multiple pregnancy.
  - Nuchal translucency (NT; see later).

SCREENING FOR DOWN'S SYNDROME

MICRO-facts

Risk factors for Down's syndrome:
- high maternal age;
- high nuchal translucency;
- high β-human chorionic gonadotrophin;
- low pregnancy-associated plasma protein A.

- All women are offered the **combined test** between 11 and 14 weeks. Three factors are tested:
  - NT on ultrasound:

- – this is the thickness of subcutaneous fluid at the back of the fetal neck.
  - Serum β-human chorionic gonadotrophin.
  - Serum pregnancy-associated plasma protein A.
- These are integrated with the maternal age to calculate the risk of Down's syndrome.
- The combined test is described as positive if the risk of Down's syndrome is greater than 1:150.
- Women with a positive result are offered pre-natal diagnosis by amniocentesis or chorionic villus sampling (CVS).
- The combined test is 75% sensitive and has a ≤3% false positive rate.

MICRO-facts

Screening for Down's syndrome: important points in counselling

Women are given a full explanation of the screening test and its implications early in the pregnancy to allow them to make an informed decision about whether to have the test. They should consider the following:

- How they would feel about having a baby with Down's syndrome.
- What they would do if the screening test was positive.
- The risk of miscarriage associated with diagnosis by chorionic villus sampling and amniocentesis.
- What action they might take if the diagnosis was positive.

MICRO-print

Beyond 14 weeks nuchal translucency cannot be measured. Between 14 and 20 weeks the **quadruple test** is used. This measures serum β-human chorionic gonadotrophin, oestriol, α-fetoprotein and inhibin A.

ANOMALY SCAN: WEEK 18–20

MICRO-facts

Approximately 1% of fetuses will have an anatomical abnormality on the scan. Spina bifida is one of the most common neural tube defects. Failure of the spinal cord to close causes a spectrum of disabilities, including lower limb paralysis and incontinence.

Obstetrics

- **Procedure**:
  - ultrasound scan.
- **Indication**:
  - Identification of fetal anomalies, including:
    - neural tube defects;
    - congenital heart defects;
    - bowel obstruction;
    - abdominal wall defects;
    - renal tract abnormalities;
    - cleft lip and palate;
    - talipes equinovarus.
  - Estimation of amniotic fluid.
  - Identification of low-lying placenta:
    - this prompts a repeat scan later in the pregnancy (at 34–36 weeks) to exclude placenta praevia.
  - Fetal measurements can be taken to establish well-being.

> **MICRO-print**
> In duodenal atresia the duodenum is a solid structure rather than a hollow tube. It is identified by polyhydramnios and a 'double bubble' appearance on the 20 week anomaly scan. In one-third of these cases the fetus also has Down's syndrome.

2.4 PRE-NATAL DIAGNOSIS

CHORIONIC VILLUS SAMPLING AND AMNIOCENTESIS

- **Indication**:
  - diagnosis of chromosomal abnormalities, e.g. Down's syndrome.
- **Timing**:
  - CVS: from 11 weeks;
  - amniocentesis: from 15 weeks.
- **Procedure**:
  - under ultrasound guidance, a fine needle is passed transabdominally;
  - in amniocentesis, amniotic fluid containing fetal fibroblasts is removed;
  - in CVS, chorionic villi are aspirated;
  - chromosomal analysis is conducted on the fetal tissue.
- **Complications**:
  - Miscarriage:
    - amniocentesis: 1%;
    - CVS: 1–2%.

- Haemorrhage.
- Infection.
- Rhesus sensitization.

2.5 PHYSIOLOGICAL CHANGES IN PREGNANCY

For the physiological changes in pregnancy, see Fig. 2.2.

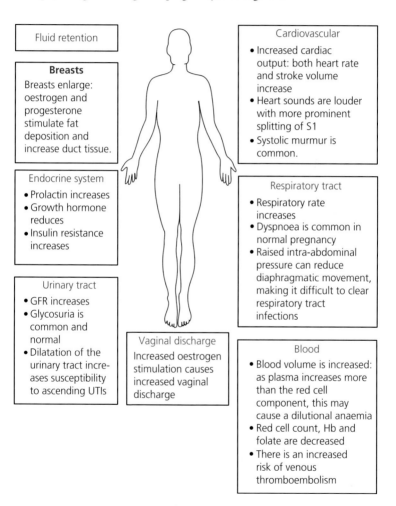

Fluid retention

Breasts

Breasts enlarge: oestrogen and progesterone stimulate fat deposition and increase duct tissue.

Endocrine system
- Prolactin increases
- Growth hormone reduces
- Insulin resistance increases

Urinary tract
- GFR increases
- Glycosuria is common and normal
- Dilatation of the urinary tract increases susceptibility to ascending UTIs

Vaginal discharge

Increased oestrogen stimulation causes increased vaginal discharge

Cardiovascular
- Increased cardiac output: both heart rate and stroke volume increase
- Heart sounds are louder with more prominent splitting of S1
- Systolic murmur is common.

Respiratory tract
- Respiratory rate increases
- Dyspnoea is common in normal pregnancy
- Raised intra-abdominal pressure can reduce diaphragmatic movement, making it difficult to clear respiratory tract infections

Blood
- Blood volume is increased: as plasma increases more than the red cell component, this may cause a dilutional anaemia
- Red cell count, Hb and folate are decreased
- There is an increased risk of venous thromboembolism

Fig. 2.2 Physiological changes in pregnancy. GFR, glomerular filtration rate; Hb, haemoglobin; UTI, urinary tract infection.

2.6 COMMON SYMPTOMS IN PREGNANCY

The following are **common complaints in pregnancy and their treatments**.

- Nausea and vomiting:
  - if severe (e.g. unable to tolerate liquids, dehydration) admit to hospital;
  - otherwise, advise rest and dietary modification (small, cold meals);
  - ginger may help.
- Heartburn:
  - modify diet;
  - adjust sleeping position: raise the head of the bed;
  - antacids.
- Backache:
  - exercise;
  - massage.
- Constipation.
  - increase dietary fibre;
  - stool softeners if needed.
- Varicose veins:
  - compression stockings improve symptoms.
- Haemorrhoids:
  - modify diet;
  - haemorrhoid creams if needed.
- Symphysis pubis dysfunction:
  - this is pain in the pubic and sacroiliac joints;
  - treatment:
    - analgesia;
    - physiotherapy.
- Itching:
  - commonly benign, but can be due to obstetric cholestasis (see Chapter 3, Medical problems in pregnancy).
- Ankle oedema:
  - commonly benign: advise raising the legs;
  - if sudden onset, exclude pre-eclampsia.
- Abdominal pain:
  - commonly benign, but do not forget surgical causes for the acute abdomen.

- Vaginal candidiasis:
    - more common in pregnancy;
    - oral treatment is contraindicated; use imidazole pessaries.
- Carpal tunnel syndrome:
    - more common owing to fluid retention;
    - wearing a wrist splint at night may help.
- Leg cramps.

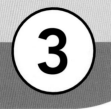

3 Medical problems in pregnancy

3.1 INTRODUCTION

The physiological changes that occur during pregnancy can affect
pre-existing medical conditions, requiring specialist management. Conversely,
pre-existing disease may complicate a pregnancy. This chapter will focus on the
following:

- endocrine conditions;
- hypertensive conditions;
- neurological conditions;
- liver conditions;
- infections and pregnancy;
- rhesus disease.

3.2 ENDOCRINE CONDITIONS

DIABETES (TYPE 1 OR 2)

- **Relevant physiological changes in pregnancy**:
  - Insulin resistance increases in pregnancy. Therefore, to maintain good
    glycaemic control, the insulin requirement may increase as the
    pregnancy progresses.
  - Falling insulin requirements in later pregnancy are a sign of impending
    placental failure.
  - Insulin requirements return to pre-pregnancy levels post-delivery very
    quickly.
- **Complications**:
  - These are due to hyperglycaemia.
  - **Maternal**:
    - Pre-eclampsia (see later under Pre-eclampsia).
    - Infection.
    - Progression of existing retinopathy.
    - Nephropathy.
    - Caesarean section/instrumental delivery.
    - Difficult labour.

MICRO-facts

Maternal glucose is able to cross the placenta and enter the fetal circulation, but maternal insulin cannot.

- **Fetal/neonatal**:
    - Congenital abnormalities:
        - ○ neural tube defects;
        - ○ heart defects.
    - Pre-term labour.
    - Reduced fetal lung maturity.
    - Macrosomia (see Fig. 3.1):
        - ○ 'large baby'.

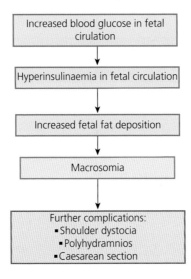

Fig. 3.1 Pathophysiology of macrosomia.

- Intra-partum complications:
    - ○ shoulder dystocia;
    - ○ fetal distress;
    - ○ sudden fetal death.
- Neonatal hypoglycaemia (see Fig. 3.2):
    - ○ particularly in the first 24 hours post-delivery.

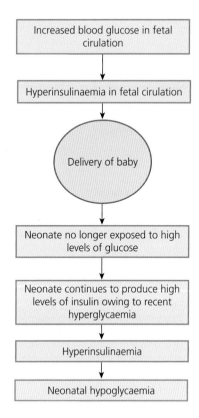

Fig. 3.2 Pathophysiology of neonatal hypoglycaemia.

- **Investigations**:
  - **Maternal**:
    – Haemoglobin A_{1C} (HbA$_{1C}$) to monitor glycaemic control.
  - **Fetal** (see Chapter 5, Fetal growth and surveillance):
    – In addition to the routine scans:
      o specialist cardiac scan;
      o serial growth scans: to monitor fetal growth and liquor volume.
- **Management**:
  - **Multidisciplinary team** (MDT): the following members should be involved:
    – obstetrician;
    – diabetes consultant;
    – midwife/nurse specialist;
    – dietician.

- **Pre-conceptual advice**:
  - diabetic women should be counselled on the importance of achieving good glycaemic control pre-conceptually and throughout their pregnancy;
  - therapeutic dose of folic acid (5 mg/day) should be prescribed to reduce the risk of neural tube defects.

MICRO-facts

The usual dose of folic acid is 0.4 mg or 400 mcg/day. For women with an increased risk of having a fetus with a neural tube defect, e.g. maternal diabetes, the dose increases to 5 mg/day.

- **Antenatal care**:
  - maintain blood glucose levels at 4–6 mmol/L;
  - encourage patients to monitor their finger-prick glucose levels;
  - use HbA_{1C} levels to monitor long-term control;
  - type 1 diabetics may need to increase their insulin dose;
  - type 2 diabetics may need to start using insulin;
  - monitor fetus as above.
- **Delivery**:
  - aim for vaginal delivery around 38 weeks' gestation;
  - fetal or maternal compromise may require earlier delivery;
  - a sliding scale of insulin and a dextrose infusion are used to maintain normoglycaemia during labour;
  - complications such as macrosomia may require a caesarean section.

GESTATIONAL DIABETES

- **Definition**:
  - development of impaired glucose tolerance during pregnancy that normalizes after pregnancy;
  - biochemical definitions vary, but generally gestational diabetes can be diagnosed if the blood glucose level is >9.0 mmol/L 2 hours after 75 g glucose load.
- **Epidemiology**:
  - affects 1–2% of pregnant women.
- **Risk factors**:
  - previous history of gestational diabetes;
  - fetus >4 kg;
  - previous unexplained stillbirth;
  - family history of diabetes;
  - high body mass index;
  - presence of polyhydramnios/persistent glycosuria.

- **Complications**:
  - see Diabetes (type 1 or 2).
- **Investigations**:
  - **Maternal**:
    - screening tests;
    - may consider if risk factors are present;
    - oral glucose tolerance test.
  - **Fetal**:
    - same as for diabetes (type 1 or 2).
- **Management**:
  - Diet control:
    - high fibre and low carbohydrates.
  - May require metformin and/or insulin.
- **Prognosis**:
  - It is estimated that 50% of women with gestational diabetes will be diagnosed with diabetes within the next 10 years.

THYROID DISEASE

- **Relevant physiological changes in pregnancy**:
  - The levels of free thyroid hormones do not change during pregnancy.
- **Complications**:
  - These may occur in poorly controlled disease.
  - **Maternal**:
    - Hypothyroidism: pre-eclampsia.
    - Hyperthyroidism: 'thyroid storm'
      - ○ severe hyperthyroidism;
      - ○ may be precipitated by stress, e.g. time of delivery.
  - **Fetal/neonatal**:
    - Hypothyroidism:
      - ○ intellectual and growth impairment during childhood; this is usually due to maternal iodine deficiency.
    - Hyperthyroidism:
      - ○ neonatal thyrotoxicosis (rare); this may occur if maternal thyroid-stimulating antibodies cross the placenta;
      - ○ tachycardia;
      - ○ prematurity;
      - ○ stillbirth.
- **Investigations**:
  - **Maternal**:
    - thyroid-stimulating hormone (TSH);
    - FT_4 and FT_3 (free thyroid hormone) levels;
    - TSH, FT_4 and FT_3 may need to be checked each trimester in women already on thyroid medication.

- **Management**:
  - **General**:
    - MDT care.
    - Regular monitoring of maternal thyroid function.
  - **Hypothyroidism**:
    - Thyroid hormone replacement with thyroxine (T_4).
    - The dose of thyroxine may need to be adjusted in pregnant women who are already taking it.
  - **Hyperthyroidism**:
    - Carbimazole or propylthiouracil:
      - The lowest therapeutic dose should be used, as both drugs can cross the placenta and may cause neonatal hypothyroidism.

3.3 HYPERTENSIVE CONDITIONS

Hypertension in pregnancy may be pre-existing or new onset, which may be in the form of either pregnancy-induced hypertension or pre-eclampsia.

PRE-EXISTING HYPERTENSION

- **Epidemiology**:
  - affects 1–3% of pregnant women.

> **MICRO-facts**
>
> Risk factors for developing superimposed pre-eclampsia:
> - renal disease;
> - diabetes;
> - blood pressure ≥160/110 mmHg before 20 weeks' gestation.

- **Changes in physiology**:
  - Blood pressure (BP) falls in the second trimester, but usually rises back to pre-pregnancy levels in the third trimester.
  - The initial fall in BP may mask any pre-existing hypertension.
- **Complications**:
  - **Maternal**:
    - Pre-eclampsia:
      - women with pre-existing hypertension are six times more likely to develop pre-eclampsia.
    - Placental abruption (see Chapter 7, Complications in labour).
    - Heart failure.
    - Intra-cerebral haemorrhage (rare).

- **Fetal/neonatal**:
  - Growth restriction:
    - due to placental insufficiency.
- **Investigations**:
  - **Maternal**:
    - Exclude secondary hypertension:
      - renal ultrasound;
      - routine blood tests;
      - echocardiogram to exclude coarctation of aorta;
      - 24 hour urine collections for vanillylmandelic acid to exclude phaeochromocytoma.
    - To prevent pre-eclampsia developing:
      - additional antenatal appointments with regular BP monitoring;
      - check for proteinuria: urine dipstick; protein–creatinine ratio; 24 hour urine protein;
      - uric acid levels;
      - Doppler ultrasound.
  - **Fetal**:
    - Serial growth scans:
      - to identify growth restriction.
- **Management**:
  - first-line: labetalol (β-blocker).
  - second-line: methyldopa (centrally acting anti-hypertensive).
  - third-line: nifedipine (calcium channel antagonist).
  - angiotensin-converting enzyme inhibitors and diuretics should be avoided because of their teratogenic effect.

PREGNANCY-INDUCED HYPERTENSION

- **Definition**:
  - new onset hypertension (>140/90 mmHg) during pregnancy, with absence of significant proteinuria and no features of pre-eclampsia.
- **Epidemiology**:
  - affects 4–8% of pregnant women.
- **Complications**:
  - see Pre-existing hypertension.
- **Investigations**:
  - **Maternal**:
    - regular BP monitoring;
    - urine dipstick for proteinuria.
- **Management**:
  - If BP >150/100 mmHg:
    - first line: labetalol;
    - second line: methyldopa.

PRE-ECLAMPSIA

- **Definition**:
  - A multisystem disorder characterized by the following:
    - hypertension (≥140/90 mmHg) recorded on two separate occasions at least 4 hours apart;
    - proteinuria ≥ 300 mg/24 hours;
    - arises after the 20th week of gestation;
    - occurs in previously normotensive women and resolves after delivery.
- **Classification**:
  - Mild:
    - 140–149 mmHg systolic and/or 90–99 mmHg diastolic reading.
  - Moderate:
    - 150–159 mmHg systolic and/or 100–109 mmHg diastolic reading.
  - Severe:
    - ≥160 mmHg systolic and/or ≥110 mmHg diastolic reading.
- **Epidemiology**:
  - affects around 6% of nulliparous women.
- **Risk factors**:
  - Nulliparity.
  - Previous history.
  - Family history:
    - risk increases three to four times if the patient is a first-degree relative of an affected woman.
  - New partner.
  - Long inter-pregnancy interval.
  - Obesity.
  - Increasing maternal age.
  - Pre-existing hypertension.
  - Pre-existing renal disease.
  - Diabetes.
  - Multiple pregnancy.
- **Pathophysiology**:
  - It is a disorder of placentation and starts at the time of implantation.
  - The exact mechanism is not fully understood, but it is generally believed that the symptoms are caused by maternal vascular endothelial cell damage (see Fig. 3.3).
  - It is probably a multisystem disorder rather than a single entity.
- **Clinical features**:
  - History:
    - Asymptomatic.
    - Headache.

Obstetrics

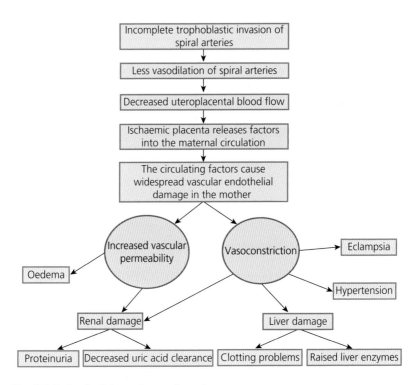

Fig. 3.3 Pathophysiology of pre-eclampsia.

- – Drowsiness.
- – Visual disturbances.
- – Epigastric pain.
- – Nausea/vomiting.
- Examination:
  - – Hypertension.
  - – Marked oedema (may be dependent or generalized).
  - – Hyper-reflexic.
  - – Clonus.
  - – Proteinuria on urinalysis:
    - ○ a positive urine dipstick for protein needs to be confirmed with a 24 hour urine sample.
- **Complications**:
  - **Maternal**:
    - – Eclampsia:
      - ○ tonic–clonic seizures, probably caused by cerebrovascular vasospasm;
      - ○ can lead to maternal/fetal hypoxia.

- Cerebrovascular haemorrhage:
  - ○ due to poor cerebral blood flow autoregulation.
- 'HELLP' syndrome:
  - ○ **H** haemolysis;
  - ○ **EL** elevated liver enzymes;
  - ○ **LP** low platelets.
- Disseminated intravascular coagulation:
  - ○ simultaneous bleeding and clotting in the circulation.
- Renal failure.
- Pulmonary oedema.
- **Fetal/neonatal**:
  - Intra-uterine growth restriction (IUGR):
    - ○ particularly if pre-eclampsia occurs <36 weeks' gestation;
    - ○ due to ischaemic placenta.
  - Pre-term delivery.
  - Placental abruption (see Chapter 7, Complications in labour)

MICRO-facts

Women with risk factors will have regular blood pressure monitoring and urinalysis.

- **Investigations**:
  - **Maternal**:
    - Diagnosis:
      - ○ urinalysis;
      - ○ urine cultures: to exclude infection;
      - ○ protein–creatinine ratio;
      - ○ 24 hour urine collection for protein;
      - ○ BP.
    - Checking for complications:
      - ○ full blood count: to assess platelet levels and haematocrit;
      - ○ urea and electrolytes: to assess renal function; urea levels should normally go down in pregnancy;
      - ○ serum uric acid levels: may be ↑ owing to renal damage; uric acid levels tend to increase with gestation;
      - ○ liver function tests (LFTs): to assess liver function; alkaline phosphatase is always raised in pregnancy;
      - ○ lactate dehydrogenase: will be ↑ in haemolysis.
  - **Fetal**:
    - Serial ultrasound scans to assess fetal growth:
      - ○ growth may be asymmetrical (head sparing).

Obstetrics

- Umbilical artery Doppler (see Chapter 5, Fetal growth and surveillance).
- Cardiotocography (CTG): to assess fetal well-being in the acute setting.
- **Management**:

MICRO-facts

Atenolol, angiotensin-converting enzyme inhibitors and angiotensin receptor blockers should be avoided because of adverse effects on the fetus.

- **Medication**:
  - Anti-hypertensives. Start if systolic BP >160 mmHg or diastolic BP >110 mmHg:
    - labetalol;
    - nifedipine;
    - hydralazine (vasodilator).
  - Magnesium sulphate:
    - treats and prevents eclampsia;
    - works by increasing cerebral perfusion and reducing cerebral oedema;
    - each unit will have its own protocol for the use of magnesium sulphate.

MICRO-print
Magnesium sulphate toxicity

Deep tendon reflexes are lost initially, and may be followed by life-threatening complications:

- respiratory depression;
- hypotension;
- renal impairment.

  - Corticosteroids:
    - should be considered before 34 weeks' gestation to encourage fetal lung maturity, providing there is time.
- **Reasons for admission**:
  - Symptomatic.
  - Proteinuria (≥ + + on urine dipstick or >300 mg/24 hours).
  - Severe hypertension (≥170/110 mmHg).
  - Fetal compromise.

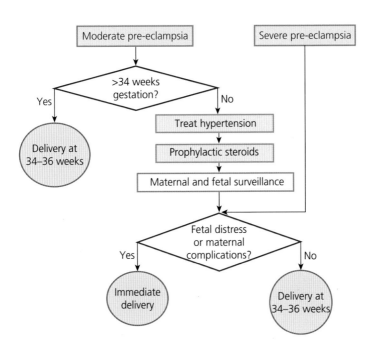

Fig. 3.4 Timing of delivery in pre-eclampsia.

- **Delivery**:
  - The timing of delivery is determined by both maternal and fetal well-being.
  - If there is mild hypertension but no fetal compromise → term delivery.
  - See Fig. 3.4.
- **Type of delivery**:
  - If <34 weeks → caesarean section may be advised.
  - If >34 weeks → consider vaginal delivery:
    - induction of labour is possible;
    - epidural analgesia will help reduce BP (see Chapter 6, Labour);
    - CTG monitoring;
    - anti-hypertensives;
    - if maternal BP >170/110 mmHg, discourage pushing during the second stage as this could lead to an intra-cerebral haemorrhage;
    - during the third stage, Syntocinon should be given;
    - ergometrine is contraindicated because it can increase BP.

MICRO-facts

Although delivery resolves the disease, the complications of pre-eclampsia can still occur postpartum. Women should be carefully reviewed before discharge from hospital.

- **Post-natal care**:
  - Continue BP treatment:
    - ○ can take up to 3 months for BP to return to normal.
  - Offer post-natal review to discuss the pregnancy.
  - Pre-conception counselling for future pregnancies.

MICRO-case

A 34-year-old woman was diagnosed with pre-eclampsia at 28 weeks' gestation following consistently high blood pressure (BP) readings at her antenatal appointments. The highest systolic reading was 180 mmHg. Her 24 hour urine collection showed 500 mg of protein. She was asymptomatic but had bilateral peripheral oedema on examination. She had no medical problems. She had a healthy 11-year-old son. Labetalol and nifedipine were started to control her BP. This treatment was continued as an outpatient, with regular maternal check-ups and fetal surveillance. The serial ultrasound scans of the fetus showed no growth restriction. She did not develop any symptoms or complications.

At 36 weeks' gestation, she was admitted for induction of labour and a normal vaginal delivery.

Key points:

- Pre-eclampsia is often asymptomatic.
- Anti-hypertensives such as labetalol and nifedipine should be started when the systolic BP is >160 mmHg.
- Once a diagnosis of pre-eclampsia is made, there is a need for regular maternal check-ups (to check for complications) and serial ultrasound scans of the fetus (to assess fetal growth).

MICRO-reference

National Collaborating Centre for Women's and Children's Health. Hypertension in pregnancy: the management of hypertensive disorders during pregnancy. NICE clinical guideline. London, UK: National Institute for Health and Clinical Excellence, 2010. Available at http://www.nice.org.uk/nicemedia/live/13098/50475/50475.pdf

Royal College of Obstetricians and Gynaecologists. The management of severe pre-eclampsia/eclampsia. Green Top Guideline no. 10(A). London, UK: RCOG, 2006. Available at http://www.rcog.org.uk/files/rcog-corp/uploaded-files/GT10aManagementPreeclampsia2006.pdf

3.4 NEUROLOGICAL CONDITIONS

EPILEPSY

- **Complications**:
  - **Maternal**:
    - Hypoxia.
    - Death.
  - **Fetal/neonatal**:
    - Complications of anti-epileptic drugs (AEDs):
      - ○ congenital abnormalities – risk doubles with AED use;
      - ○ developmental delay;
      - ○ growth restriction.
    - Complications of maternal seizures:
      - ○ fetal hypoxia.
- **Investigations**:
  - **Fetal**:
    - a specialist cardiac scan in addition to the routine scans.
- **Management**:
  - **Pre-conceptual advice**:
    - epilepsy should be controlled with the lowest possible therapeutic dose of AEDs;
    - therapeutic dose of folic acid (5 mg/day) should be prescribed and continued throughout the pregnancy.
  - **Antenatal care**:
    - AEDs should be continued;
    - consider increasing the dose of AEDs if seizures are poorly controlled.

MICRO-facts

Poor seizure control is potentially more harmful to the fetus than the side-effects of AEDs.

- **Neonatal care**:
  - Vitamin K injections:
    - ○ the maternal use of AEDs in pregnancy results in a fetal deficiency of vitamin K-dependent clotting factors.

Obstetrics

3.5 LIVER CONDITIONS

OBSTETRIC CHOLESTASIS

- **Definition**:
    - A condition acquired during pregnancy in which bile flow out of the liver is reduced, resulting in a build-up of bile acids in the circulation.
    - It is characterized by the following features:
        - pruritus without a skin rash (especially affecting the palms and soles of the feet);
        - abnormal LFTs;
        - no alternative causes for the features above;
        - features resolve post-delivery.
- **Epidemiology**:
    - affects 0.7% of pregnancies.
- **Risk factors**:
    - Asian origin;
    - previous history;
    - family history.
- **Pathophysiology**:
    - The exact mechanism remains unclear but increased sensitivity to the cholestatic effects of oestrogen and environmental and genetic factors may have a role.
- **Clinical features**:
    - **Maternal**:
        - pruritus;
        - scratch marks;
        - pale stools;
        - steatorrhoea;
        - dark urine.

MICRO-facts

Itching typically occurs on the hands and the feet.
Jaundice is surprisingly uncommon in obstetric cholestasis.

- **Fetal**:
    - arrhythmias.

- **Complications**:
  - **Maternal**:
    - severe pruritus;
    - sleep deprivation.
  - **Fetal/neonatal**:
    - arrhythmias;
    - pre-term delivery;
    - stillbirth.
- **Investigations**:
  - **Maternal**:
    - LFTs.
    - Viral serology:
      - ○ to exclude other causes of abnormal LFTs.
    - Liver ultrasound.
  - **Fetal**:
    - The fetus is often not monitored since there is no accurate method for predicting adverse events.
    - Some obstetricians do serial ultrasound scans and weekly or twice-weekly Doppler scans.
- **Management**:
  - Induction of labour at 37 weeks' gestation is usually recommended owing to the unpredictable nature of the disease.
  - Ursodeoxycholic acid:
    - may help relieve itching but is not licensed for use in pregnancy.
  - Water-soluble vitamin K:
    - cholestasis can reduce vitamin K absorption, increasing the risk of postpartum haemorrhage.
- **Prognosis**:
  - Pruritus and abnormal LFTs should resolve post-delivery.
  - There is a high recurrence rate.
  - Family members will have a higher risk of developing the condition.

MICRO-reference

Royal College of Obstetricians and Gynaecologists. Obstetric cholestasis. Green Top Guideline no. 43. London, UK: RCOG, 2006. Available at http://www.rcog.org.uk/files/rcog-corp/uploaded-files/GT43Obstetric Cholestasis2006.pdf

Obstetrics

Table 3.1 Comparison of complications.

DISEASE	MATERNAL COMPLICATIONS	FETAL/NEONATAL COMPLICATIONS
Diabetes	Pre-eclampsia Infection Retinopathy Nephropathy Caesarean section Instrumental delivery Difficult labour	Congenital abnormalities Pre-term labour ↑ fetal lung maturity Macrosomia Shoulder dystocia Fetal distress Sudden fetal death Neonatal hypoglycaemia
Hyperthyroidism	'Thyroid storm'	Neonatal thyrotoxicosis Tachycardia Prematurity Stillbirth
Hypothyroidism	Pre-eclampsia	Intellectual impairment Growth impairment
Hypertension	Pre-eclampsia Placental abruption Heart failure Intra-cerebral haemorrhage	Growth restriction
Pre-eclampsia	Eclampsia Cerebrovascular haemorrhage 'HELLP' syndrome DIC Renal failure Pulmonary oedema	IUGR Pre-term delivery Placental abruption
Epilepsy	Hypoxia Death	Congenitalabnormalities Developmental delay Growth restriction Fetal hypoxia
Obstetric cholestasis	Severe pruritus Sleep deprivation	Arrhythmias Pre-term delivery Stillbirth

DIC, disseminated intravascular coagulation; HELLP, haemolysis, elevated liver enzymes and low platelets; IUGR, intra-uterine growth restriction.

Obstetrics

3.6 INFECTIONS AND PREGNANCY

This section will focus on the TORCH infections and group B streptococcal infection. The potential complications of hepatitis B, human immunodeficiency virus and syphilis have been included in Table 3.2. The following infections are not featured in this section but are also important:

- parvovirus;
- listeriosis;
- malaria;
- gonorrhoea (see Chapter 19, Genital tract infections);
- *Chlamydia* (see Chapter 19, Genital tract infections);
- bacterial vaginosis (see Chapter 19, Genital tract infections).

MICRO-facts

TORCH infections

You may see this acronym used on maternity units. It stands for the following:

- **TO** Toxoplasmosis.
- **R** Rubella.
- **C** Cytomegalovirus.
- **H** Herpesviruses.

These infections can cause congenital abnormalities.

TOXOPLASMOSIS

- **Epidemiology**:
  - affects 0.2% of pregnant women in the UK.
- **Pathology**:
  - caused by the protozoan *Toxoplasma gondii*;
  - this is found in cat faeces or infected meat.
- **Clinical features**:
  - asymptomatic;
  - fever;
  - sore throat;
  - malaise;
  - headache.
- **Complications**:
  - Early maternal infection tends to result in more severe fetal damage.
  - **Maternal**:
    - fulminating pneumonitis;

  - encephalomyelitis;
  - brain abscesses (in acquired immunodeficiency syndrome).
 - **Fetal/neonatal**:
   - hydrocephalus;
   - microcephaly;
   - chorioretinitis;
   - convulsions;
   - cerebral calcifications.
- **Diagnosis**:
  - **Maternal**:
    - Test for immunoglobulin M.
  - **Fetal**:
    - Ultrasound:
      ○ to identify hydrocephalus.
    - Amniocentesis.
- **Management**:
  - **Maternal**:
    - Spiramycin.
    - Health education to prevent infection:
      ○ avoid eating/handling raw meat;
      ○ avoid handling cats and cat litter;
      ○ frequent handwashing with soap and water.
  - **Neonatal**:
    - Pyrimethamine and sulphonamide.

RUBELLA

- **Epidemiology**:
  - rare due to childhood vaccination programme.
- **Pathology**:
  - caused by rubella virus.
- **Clinical features**:
  - fever;
  - painful joints;
  - sore throat;
  - macular rash.
- **Complications**:
  - Higher risk of developing complications if infected in early pregnancy.
  - **Fetal/neonatal**:
    - cardiovascular defects;
    - eye defects;
    - deafness;
    - microcephaly;
    - hepatitis;

- thrombocytopenia;
- pre-term birth.
- **Diagnosis**:
  - Maternal antibody levels (done at booking visit).
  - Congenital infection:
    - isolate virus from urine or faeces.
- **Management**:
  - Non-immune and pregnant women → advised to avoid known cases of rubella.
  - Women who are non-immune and not pregnant → MMR (measles, mumps and rubella) vaccine.
    - As this is a live, attenuated vaccine, women are advised against becoming pregnant for 3 months after the vaccination and should use contraception during this time.
  - If maternal antibody levels are low → booster vaccination after delivery.
  - If maternal infection confirmed → offer termination if <16 weeks' gestation.

CYTOMEGALOVIRUS

- **Epidemiology**:
  - affects up to 1:200 pregnancies.
- **Pathology**:
  - Cytomegalovirus (CMV) is a herpesvirus that is spread through respiratory and genitourinary tracts.
  - Maternal infection is often asymptomatic.
- **Clinical features**:
  - asymptomatic;
  - non-specific features.
- **Complications**:
  - Vertical transmission occurs in around 40% of affected pregnancies.
  - About 10% of infected neonates show symptoms.
  - Fetal/neonatal:
    - microcephaly;
    - blindness;
    - deafness;
    - IUGR;
    - thrombocytopenia;
    - pneumonitis.
- **Diagnosis**:
  - Routine ultrasound scans:
    - may show abnormalities.

- Maternal CMV antibodies.
- If maternal infection → amniocentesis to check for vertical transmission.
- **Management**:
  - Anti-viral drugs for CMV cannot be used in pregnancy.
  - The woman may choose to have a termination of pregnancy.

VARICELLA ZOSTER ('CHICKENPOX')

- **Epidemiology**:
  - Chickenpox occurs in 0.05% of pregnancies.
- **Pathology**:
  - Primary infection with varicella zoster causes maternal chickenpox.
  - Subsequently, the virus lies dormant in the sensory root ganglia of the spinal cord.
  - Reactivation of the virus causes shingles.
- **Complications**:
  - **Fetal/neonatal**:
    - Birth defects (1–2%).
    - Severe neonatal infection:
      - may occur if there is maternal infection in the 4 weeks before delivery.
    - Fetal varicella syndrome.

MICRO-print

Fetal varicella syndrome

- This may occur if maternal infection develops before 20 weeks' gestation. Features include:
  - skin scarring;
  - eye defects;
  - neurological abnormalities (dysfunction of bowel and bladder).

- **Diagnosis**:
  - often clinical.
- **Management**:
  - **Maternal**:
    - Aciclovir is used to treat infection.
    - Prophylactic immunoglobulin should be considered for women who have had recent exposure to chickenpox or shingles and lack immunity to varicella zoster virus on serological studies.

- **Fetal/neonatal**:
  - Give prophylactic immunoglobulin to neonates delivered in the period 2 days before to 5 days after the onset of maternal symptoms.
  - Aciclovir for confirmed infection.

> **MICRO-reference**
> Royal College of Obstetricians and Gynaecologists. Chickenpox in pregnancy. Green Top Guideline no. 13. London, UK: RCOG, 2007. Available at http://www.rcog.org.uk/files/rcog-corp/uploaded-files/GT13ChickenpoxinPregnancy2007.pdf

HERPES SIMPLEX (GENITAL HERPES)

- **Epidemiology**:
  - <5% of pregnant women have prior herpes simplex infection.
- **Pathology**:
  - Genital herpes is usually caused by herpes simplex virus type 2 (HSV-2) but can be caused by herpes simplex virus type 1 (HSV-1).
- **Clinical features**:
  - painful ulcers around the introitus;
  - dysuria;
  - local lymphadenopathy.
- **Complications**:
  - **Fetal/neonatal**:
    - Neonatal infection (rare):
      - ○ damage to skin/eyes/mouth/multiple organs;
      - ○ high mortality rate;
      - ○ the risk of neonatal infection is higher with primary genital herpes than with recurrent genital herpes.
- **Diagnosis**:
  - viral swab of lesions;
  - HSV antibody testing is used to differentiate between primary and recurrent infection.
- **Management**:
  - refer to genitourinary medicine;
  - caesarean section may be advised for women who deliver within 6 weeks of a primary infection or who have primary active genital vesicles at the time of delivery;
  - aciclovir is used to treat the mother and neonate.

Obstetrics

GROUP B *STREPTOCOCCUS*

- **Epidemiology**:
  - 25% women are carriers.
- **Pathology**:
  - The group B *Streptococcus* (GBS) *Streptococcus agalactiae* is carried in the gut and genital tract of women.
  - It causes **no** maternal symptoms but may be transmitted to the neonate at delivery.
- **Risk factors for GBS infection in neonates**:
  - previous baby affected by GBS;
  - GBS detected in the urine during current pregnancy.
  - pre-term labour;
  - prolonged rupture of membranes (>18 hours);
  - intra-partum fever (>38°C).
- **Complications**:
  - **Fetal/perinatal/neonatal**:
    - Neonatal GBS infection:
      - septicaemia;
      - pneumonia;
      - meningitis.
- **Diagnosis**:
  - vaginal/rectal swabs.
- **Management**:
  - routine screening is not recommended;
  - if GBS is detected incidentally → consider intra-partum penicillin prophylaxis;
  - if previous baby affected by GBS infection → offer intra-partum penicillin prophylaxis;
  - use clindamycin if the woman is allergic to penicillin.

Table 3.2 Fetal/neonatal complications of infections during pregnancy.

INFECTION	FETAL/NEONATAL COMPLICATIONS
Toxoplasmosis	Hydrocephalus
	Microcephaly
	Chorioretinitis
	Convulsions
	Cerebral calcifications
Rubella	Cardiovascular defects
	Eye defects
	Deafness
	Microcephaly
	Hepatitis
	Thrombocytopenia
	Pre-term birth
Cytomegalovirus	Microcephaly
	Blindness
	Deafness
	IUGR
	Thrombocytopenia
	Pneumonitis
Varicella zoster virus	Birth defects
	Severe neonatal infection
	Fetal varicella syndrome
Herpes simplex virus	Neonatal infection leading to damage to skin/eyes/mouth/multiple organs
Group B *Streptococcus*	Neonatal infection leading to septicaemia/pneumonia/meningitis
Hepatitis B	Vertical transmission with 90% of infected neonates becoming chronic carriers
HIV	Vertical transmission
	Stillbirth
	Pre-eclampsia
	IUGR
	Prematurity

Obstetrics

INFECTION	FETAL/NEONATAL COMPLICATIONS
Syphilis	Miscarriage
	Stillbirth
	Congenital syphilis (rash, hepatitis, splenomegaly, neurosyphilis, sensorineural deafness)

HIV, human immunodeficiency virus; IUGR, intra-uterine growth restriction.

3.7 RHESUS DISEASE

- **Definition**:
    - Rhesus disease is a form of red cell iso-immunization, in which a mother's immune system attacks antigens found on fetal blood cells that enter her circulation.
- **Background**:
    - Blood can be classified by the rhesus system (C, D and E antigens).
    - Of these, the D antigen is the most important.
    - If a person is 'D rhesus positive', their red blood cells will express the D antigen.
    - If a person is 'D rhesus negative', their red blood cells will not display the D antigen. These people will produce antibodies against D antigen if they are exposed to it (sensitization).
- **Pathophysiology**:
    - see Fig. 3.5.

MICRO-facts

Potential sensitizing events
- Termination of pregnancy
- Miscarriage
- Ectopic pregnancy
- Intra-uterine death
- Antepartum haemorrhage
- External cephalic version
- Invasive uterine procedure (amniocentesis or chorionic villus sampling)
- Delivery
- Maternal trauma

From Impey L, Child T. Obstetrics and gynaecology, 3rd edn. Oxford, UK: Wiley-Blackwell, 2008.

- **Clinical features of rhesus disease**:
    - Neonatal jaundice.

Obstetrics

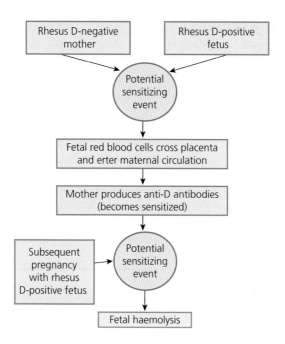

Fig. 3.5 **Pathophysiology of rhesus disease.**

- Neonatal anaemia (haemolytic disease of the newborn).
- *In utero* anaemia:
  - can lead to fetal cardiac failure, ascites, hydrops (oedema) and death.

MICRO-facts

The first pregnancy causes sensitization but is not affected.

- **Investigations**:
  - Mother:
    - booking visit: rhesus status and test for maternal anti-D antibodies;
    - after delivery: maternal anti-D antibody check and Kleihauer test.

MICRO-facts

If maternal anti-D antibodies are detected, giving anti-D will be useless as the mother is already sensitized. In these cases, more prudent monitoring is needed.

Obstetrics

- Fetus:
  - Doppler ultrasounds and fetal blood sampling to check for fetal anaemia;
  - after delivery: test cord blood for rhesus status, blood group, haemoglobin, bilirubin and Coombs' test.
- **Prevention and management**:
  - Mother:
    - If rhesus negative, give anti-D at 28 and 34 weeks. Also, give after any bleeding or potential sensitizing event. Anti-D will bind to any D antigens present and prevent maternal sensitization.
    - If the baby is rhesus positive, anti-D should be given after delivery. The amount given is guided by the Kleihauer test.
  - Fetus:
    - If severely anaemic, may need *in utero* or post-delivery blood transfusion.

MICRO-print

- **Kleihauer test**: detects the presence of fetal blood cells in maternal circulation.
- **Direct Coombs' test**: detects antibodies that are attached to fetal red cells (agglutination = positive test).
- **Indirect Coombs' test**: detects unbound antibodies (agglutination = positive test).

Other antigens involved with red cell iso-immunization include Kell and Duffy.

MICRO-reference

Royal College of Obstetricians and Gynaecologists. The use of anti-D immunoglobulin for rhesus D prophylaxis. Green Top Guideline no. 22. London, UK: RCOG, 2011. Available at http://www.rcog.org.uk/files/rcog-corp/GTG22AntiD.pdf

Obstetrics

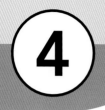

4 Multiple pregnancy

- **Epidemiology**:
  - Multiple pregnancies accounted for 1.6% of pregnancies in 2008 in England and Wales.
  - Multiple births account for 3% live births.
  - The incidence of multiple pregnancy is rising because of *in vitro* fertilization (IVF) and assisted conception.
- **Aetiology**:
  - Risk factors:
    - Assisted reproduction technology, particularly IVF, in the developed world:
      - ○ no more than two embryos can be transferred into the uterus: this is mandatory in the UK;
      - ○ up to 24% of successful cases of IVF result in multiple pregnancy.
    - Previous history of twins.
    - Increasing maternal age.
    - Increasing parity.
    - Family history of dizygotic twins.

> **MICRO-reference**
> National Institute for Health and Clinical Excellence. Multiple pregnancy: pre-publication check–draft full guideline. London, UK: NICE, 2011. Available from http://www.nice.org.uk/guidance/index.jsp?action = download&o =55254

- **Types of twin pregnancy**:
  - Dizygotic:
    - account for 70% of twin pregnancies;
    - definition: two sperms fertilize two ova;

- the twins are non-identical;
- they always have separate placentas and amniotic sacs;
- they are dichorionic and diamniotic.
- Monozygotic:
  - account for 30% of twin pregnancies;
  - one sperm fertilizes one ovum, this then undergoes mitotic division;
  - two identical zygotes are formed;
  - the timing of the mitotic division determines whether the placenta and amniotic sac are shared or not (see Table 4.1).

Table 4.1 Types of monozygotic twins.

TYPE	FEATURES
Dichorionic, diamniotic (DCDA)	Division day 1–3
	Separate placentas and amniotic sacs
Monochorionic, diamniotic (MCDA)	Division day 4–8
	Shared placenta
	Separate amniotic sacs
Monochorionic, monoamniotic (MCMA)	Division day 9–13
	Shared placenta
	Shared amniotic sac
Conjoined	> 13 days post-fertilization
	Incomplete division
	Very rare

- **Clinical features**:
  - Can be divided into early and late pregnancy features:
    - Early pregnancy features:
      - hyperemesis;
      - uterus large for dates.
    - Late pregnancy features:
      - polyhydramnios;
      - > 2 fetal poles palpable;
      - two fetal heart rates may be audible.

- **Complications**:
    - Pre-term delivery. This is the major cause of perinatal morbidity and mortality.

MICRO-facts

Twin–twin transfusion syndrome

- It is seen almost exclusively in monochorionic twins.
- Vascular anastomoses in the shared placenta result in unequal blood distribution.
- One twin ('the donor') becomes anaemic and growth restricted.
- The other twin ('the recipient') becomes polycythaemic and may develop cardiac failure, which can eventually result in the development of hydrops.
- Perinatal mortality is very high.
- In early severe cases, laser ablation of placental vascular anastomoses can be carried out in highly specialized centres.

- Most obstetric complications are increased in multiple pregnancies. These are summarized in Table 4.2.
- The risk of complications is greater with triplets than with twins, and so on with the number of fetuses.

Table 4.2 Obstetric complications occurring in multiple pregnancies.

DURING PREGNANCY	FETAL	DURING LABOUR
Polyhydramnios	Increased perinatal mortality	Malpresentation
Pre-eclampsia	Prematurity	Postpartum haemorrhage
Anaemia	Growth restriction and fetal distress	Cord prolapse and entanglement
Antepartum haemorrhage	Twin–twin transfusion syndrome (only in monochorionic twins)	
Miscarriage	Congenital abnormalities	

- **Management**:
  - **General principles**:
    - Multiple pregnancies should be considered 'high risk'.
    - Ultrasound is used to diagnose multiple pregnancy and monitor fetal growth monthly.
    - Iron and folate supplements are required.
    - In the case of triplets or higher order pregnancy, selective reduction to a twin pregnancy may be offered; this reduces the risk of premature delivery.
  - **Intra-partum management**:
    - Vaginal delivery is acceptable provided the presentation of the first fetus is cephalic. This is regardless of the lie or presentation of the second twin.
    - Indications for caesarean section:
      - the lie of the first fetus is breech or transverse;
      - triplets.
    - The first fetus is delivered normally.
    - Continuous cardiotocography monitoring is required to identify hypoxia.
    - To deliver the second fetus successfully the following is considered:
      - external cephalic version: if the lie is abnormal;
      - internal podalic version may be undertaken if external cephalic version is unsuccessful;
      - a fetal foot is identified and then gently pulled into the birth canal;
      - administration of oxytocin prior to delivery: contractions may decrease following delivery of the first twin;
      - oxytocin intravenously post-delivery to prevent postpartum haemorrhage;
      - there is an increased likelihood of instrumental and operative delivery for the second twin, particularly if fetal distress or cord prolapse occurs.
    - Delivery of the second twin usually occurs within 20 minutes of the first.

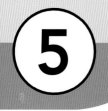

Fetal growth and surveillance

5.1 FETAL MONITORING

- **General principles**:
    - The aim of fetal monitoring is to detect abnormalities in fetal growth during pregnancy, and to identify fetal distress during labour.
    - This enables timely intervention and thus reduces perinatal morbidity and mortality.
    - The fetus is monitored in all pregnancies with standard antenatal care.
    - High-risk pregnancies require additional fetal monitoring. These are identified by maternal or fetal factors (see Table 5.1).

Table 5.1 Indications for fetal monitoring.

MATERNAL FACTORS	FETAL FACTORS
Age < 18 or > 40	Small-for-dates baby
Pre-existing disease, e.g. cardiac, renal, endocrine	Exposure to infection
	Exposure to illicit drugs
Extremes of BMI	Excess maternal alcohol
Previous obstetric complications, e.g. recurrent miscarriage, pre-eclampsia, stillbirth	
Current obstetric complications, e.g. hypertension and vaginal bleeding	
History of thrombophilia	

BMI, body mass index.

- **Indications for fetal monitoring**:
    - see Table 5.1.
- **Common methods of fetal monitoring**:
    - Doppler;
    - ultrasound;
    - biophysical profile;

- auscultation;
- cardiotocography (CTG);
- fetal scalp blood sampling.

Table 5.2 Terminology.

TERM	DEFINITION
Fetal distress	Hypoxia, which may be acute or chronic, resulting in fetal acidosis. If not reversed, it results in fetal death
Fetal compromise	A chronic situation arising from suboptimal conditions for growth and neurological development
Small for dates	The fetus or infant is below the 10th centile for estimated fetal weight or post-natal birthweight
Intra-uterine growth restriction	Failure of the fetus to reach its expected growth potential
Symmetrical growth restriction	Fetal head and abdomen circumference are proportionally small
Asymmetrical growth restriction	The fetal head circumference is large compared with the abdominal circumference. The result of placental insufficiency

DOPPLER

- **Procedure**:
  - resistance in the umbilical vessels is measured and recorded as velocity waveforms;
  - used to assess umbilical artery circulation;
  - fetal circulation can also be assessed.
- **Interpretation of results**:
  - reduced flow during diastole suggests placental dysfunction;
  - the baby may be acidotic and hypoxic.
- **Advantages**:
  - effective in detecting a growth-restricted fetus.
- **Disadvantages**:
  - does not reduce perinatal mortality in low-risk pregnancies;
  - there is insufficient evidence that assessing fetal circulation reduces perinatal mortality.

ULTRASOUND

- **Procedure**:
  - measurement of the fetal abdomen and head circumference after the first trimester.
- **Interpretation of results**:
  - the rate of growth is calculated from serial scans performed at least 2 weeks apart;
  - growth restriction is identified as symmetrical or asymmetrical.
- **Advantages**:
  - ultrasound is safe and can confirm consistent growth.
- **Disadvantages**:
  - operator inaccuracies can occur.

BIOPHYSICAL PROFILE

- **Procedure**:
  - Assesses five different fetal parameters during a 30 minute ultrasound of the fetus:
    - heart rate variability;
    - limb movement;
    - tone;
    - breathing movement;
    - amniotic fluid volume.
- **Interpretation of results**:
  - Each of the variables is scored out of 2, according to specific criteria.
  - A score of 8–10 is reassuring whereas a score below 4 is suggestive of severe compromise.
  - Changes in these variables identify the central nervous system depression that occurs with chronic hypoxia.
- **Advantages**:
  - The score is a useful guide as to when intervention may be required.
- **Disadvantages**:
  - time-consuming;
  - little value in low-risk pregnancies.

INTERMITTENT AUSCULTATION

- **Procedure**:
  - Pinard stethoscope or Doppler is used to auscultate the fetal heart rate (FHR) at the end of contractions.
- **Interpretation of results**:
  - The presence of decelerations (see Table 5.3) following a contraction indicates fetal compromise and CTG is required.

Obstetrics

- **Advantages**:
  - simple;
  - best method of assessment in low-risk pregnancies.
- **Disadvantages**:
  - over-predicts fetal distress.

CARDIOTOCOGRAPHY

- **Procedure**:
  - Transducers are placed on the abdomen or fetal scalp allowing electronic measurement of the fetal heart rate.
  - An additional transducer is used to measure uterine contractions.
  - Continuous CTG monitoring during labour is limited to high-risk cases.
- **Indications for continuous CTG monitoring in labour**:
  - meconium-stained liquor;
  - FHR <110 or >160 b.p.m.;
  - decelerations after a contraction;
  - maternal pyrexia ($38.0°C$ once or $37.5°C$ twice 2 hours apart);
  - fresh bleeding;
  - use of oxytocin for augmentation.

MICRO-reference

National Institute for Health and Clinical Excellence. Intrapartum care: quick reference guide. NICE Clinical Guidance 55. London, UK: NICE, 2010. Available at http://guidance.nice.org.uk/CG55/QuickRefGuide/pdf/English.

- **Interpretation of results**:
  - The parameters measured are used to detect fetal compromise (see Table 5.3).
  - If CTG suggests fetal hypoxia then a fetal scalp pH may be required, which may depend on the stage of labour;
  - See Fig. 5.1 for an example of a normal cardiotocograph.
- **Advantages**:
  - sensitive for the detection of fetal hypoxia.
- **Disadvantages**:
  - needs to be done every day in a high-risk patient.

Table 5.3 Cardiotocography features.

FEATURE	DEFINITION	WHAT IS NORMAL?	CAUSES OF ABNORMAL FEATURE
Baseline FHR	Mean level of a stable FHR over 5–10 minutes. Described in b.p.m.	110–150 b.p.m.	Tachycardia: >160 is associated with maternal fever, fetal infection and fetal hypoxia. Bradycardia: <100 is suggestive of fetal distress if the decline is rapid and does not improve
Baseline variability	The difference in b.p.m. between the highest FHR and the lowest over 1 minute	Variation in heart rate should be >5 b.p.m.	Variability may be <5 b.p.m. if the fetus is sleeping (this should not last for longer than 5 seconds however). Drugs (e.g. morphine) and hypoxia may also cause reduced variability
Accelerations	An increase in FHR that coincides with a contraction	An increase of ≥15 b.p.m. for >15 seconds	The absence of accelerations in an otherwise normal trace is of uncertain significance
Decelerations	A decrease in FHR	A decrease of ≥15 b.p.m. for >15 seconds	'Early decelerations' coincide with a contraction and are a normal response to fetal head compression.

(Continued)

Obstetrics

Table 5.3 (*Continued*)

FEATURE	DEFINITION	WHAT IS NORMAL?	CAUSES OF ABNORMAL FEATURE
			'Variable decelerations' vary in timing and degrees and suggest umbilical cord compression. Late decelerations continuing after the contraction signify fetal hypoxia

FHR, fetal heart rate.

FETAL SCALP BLOOD SAMPLING

- **Procedure**:
  - a small cut is made in the fetal scalp using a small blade;
  - a metal tube called an amnioscope provides access to the scalp;
  - blood is collected in a capillary tube;
  - the blood is analysed for pH and base excess.
- **Interpretation of results**:
  - A pH <7.2 signifies severe fetal hypoxia and implies immediate delivery is required.
  - If the pH value is between 7.2 and 7.25 it should be repeated in 1 hour.
  - A pH above 7.25 is normal and future action is dependent on the CTG and course of labour.
- **Advantages**:
  - a direct measure of fetal hypoxia.
- **Disadvantages**:
  - uncomfortable for the mother;
  - requires the membranes to be ruptured and the cervix to be sufficiently dilated.

5.2 MANAGING ABNORMALITIES

FETAL DISTRESS

- **Definition**:
  - an indication of fetal hypoxia and may result in fetal damage or death if not reversed.

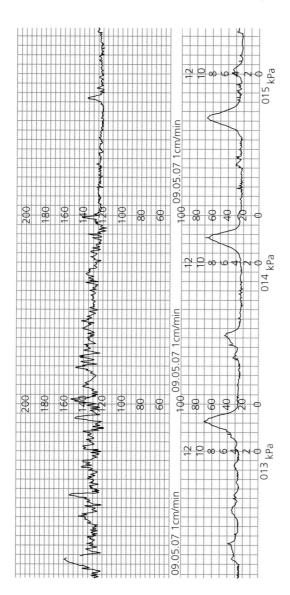

Fig. 5.1 A normal cardiotocograph, showing a baseline fetal heart rate of approximately 120 b.p.m., frequent accelerations, baseline variability of 10–15 b.p.m. and no decelerations. The uterus is contracting approximately once every 5 minutes.

- **Aetiology**:
    - poorly understood;
    - may occur as a result of reduced blood flow through the umbilical cord and placenta during maternal contractions, particularly if they are prolonged.
- **Indicative features**:
    - presence of undiluted meconium (fetal bowel contents which stain the amniotic fluid) during early labour;
    - fetal tachycardia detected on auscultation;
    - abnormal CTG patterns;
    - fetal acidosis detected by fetal scalp blood sampling.
- **Management**:
    - fetal scalp blood pH <7.2 necessitates delivery by the safest and most timely route.

SMALL-FOR-DATES AND GROWTH-RESTRICTED FETUSES

- **Definition**:
    - see Table 5.2.
- **Management**:
    - Fig. 5.2 summarizes the process involved in identification and management of small-for-dates and growth-restricted fetuses.

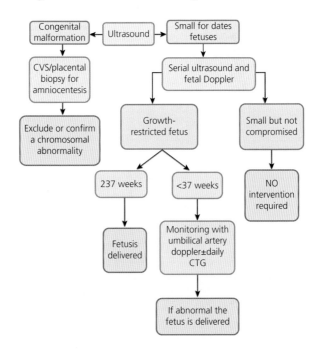

Fig. 5.2 Algorithm for the management of small-for-dates and growth-restricted fetuses. CTG, cardiotocograph; CVS, chorionic villus sampling.

MICRO-facts

Growth-restricted fetuses are at an increased risk of becoming hypoxic; therefore, it is essential to monitor them closely during pregnancy and labour.

5.3 STILLBIRTH

MICRO-facts

Fetal monitoring aims to prevent stillbirth.

- **Definition**:
  - delivery of a dead baby after 24 weeks' gestation.
- **Aetiology**:
  - unexplained in the majority of cases;
  - more common in high-risk pregnancies (see Table 5.1).
- **Clinical features**:
  - Absent fetal movements.
  - Absent heart sounds on auscultation.
  - There may be symptoms relating to the cause:
    - vaginal bleeding;
    - abdominal pain.
- **Investigations**:
  - Ultrasound scan:
    - no fetal movement, e.g. heart beat.
- **Management**:
  - If the death is associated with maternal disease, the mother is resuscitated and stabilized.
  - Labour is usually induced with prostaglandins.
  - Anti-D is given to rhesus-negative women.
  - It is essential to support the parents – they are encouraged to hold and name the baby as this can help with the grieving process.
  - A certificate of stillbirth is issued and must be taken by the parents to the Registrar of Births, Marriages and Deaths within 42 days.
  - The parents should be counselled about how helpful a post-mortem may be and any further investigations that may be useful in trying to identify a cause.
  - Bereavement counselling should be considered.

6 Labour

6.1 INTRODUCTION

This chapter describes labour for a fetus with cephalic presentation. See Chapter 7, Complications in labour for malpresentations.

- **Definition**:
  - Labour is the process by which the fetus and placenta are expelled from the uterus. This is achieved by regular, painful uterine contractions with dilatation and effacement of the cervix.
- **The fetal skull (see Fig. 6.1)**:
  - The bony plates of the fetal skull are not fused.
  - There are two soft spots or **fontanelles** between the bones.
  - These allow the bones to flex and overlap during labour.
- **Orientation of the fetal head**:
  - The part of the head that travels through the pelvis first is called the **presenting part (see Fig. 6.2)**.
  - The presenting part is determined by how much the head is flexed: the **attitude** of the head.
  - Delivery is easiest when the smallest part of the head passes through the pelvis first. This is a **vertex presentation**.
  - If the head is extended there will be a **brow** or **face** presentation.
  - The **position** of the head describes how it is rotated within the pelvis, with reference to the occiput:
    - occiput anterior (OA);
    - occiput posterior (OP);
    - occiput transverse (OT).

MICRO-facts

The optimum orientation of the fetal head for delivery is fully flexed, i.e. **vertex** presentation and **occiput anterior**. This presents the narrowest diameter.

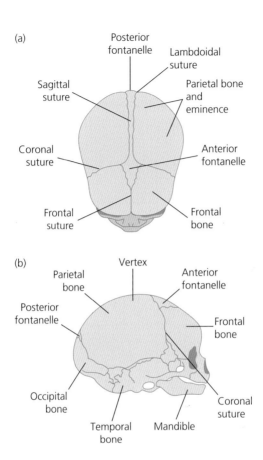

Fig. 6.1 The fetal skull from (a) superior and (b) lateral views.

Table 6.1 Summary of labour terminology.

	DEFINITIONS	TYPES
Attitude	The degree of flexion of the fetal head	Flexed Extended Hyperextended
Presenting part	The lowest part of the fetus palpable on vaginal examination	Vertex Brow Face
Position	The rotation of the head within the pelvis, using the occiput as the point of reference	Occiput anterior Occiput posterior Occiput transverse

Obstetrics

	Flexed			Extended
Attitude	Well flexed	Less well flexed (partially extended) or deflexed	Extended 'brow presentation'	Hyperextended 'face presentation'
Diameter	Suboccipito-bregmatic	Occipito-frontal	Occipito-mental	Submento-bregmatic
Measurement	9.5 cm	11.5 cm	13.0 cm	9.5 cm

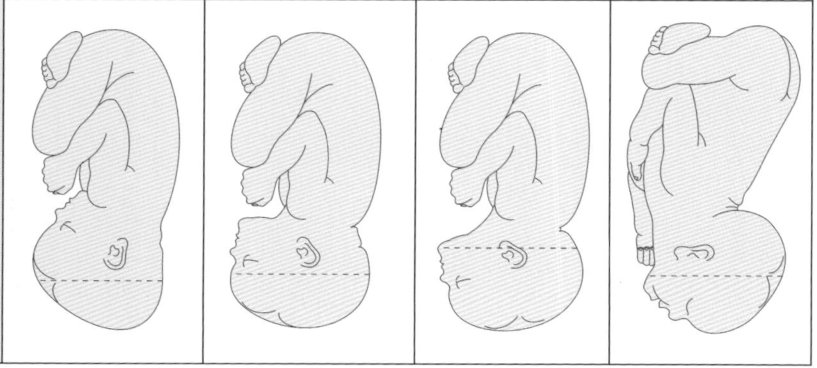

Fig. 6.2 Attitude and presentation. The attitude of the fetal head determines the presenting part, and the ease of vaginal delivery.

6.2 THE PROCESS OF NORMAL LABOUR

MICRO-facts
Regular contractions occur every 2–4 minutes, each lasting 50–60 seconds.

- **Diagnosis of labour**:
  - This is made when there are:
    - painful, regular contractions;
    - effacement and dilatation of the cervix;
    - descent of the presenting part.
- **Onset of labour**:
  - The precise trigger for the onset of labour is unknown, although prostaglandins play an important role.
  - Prostaglandins increase oxytocin release.
  - Oxytocin stimulates uterine contractions.
  - Contractions lead to effacement and dilatation of the cervix.
  - **Effacement**:
    - the pre-labour cervix is a tubular shape (see Fig. 6.3a);
    - prostaglandin release softens the cervix, which then shortens and is drawn up to be continuous with the lower segment of the uterus (see Fig. 6.3b);
    - effacement may be accompanied by the loss of a mucus plug or 'show' from the cervix.
  - **Rupture of membranes**:
    - rupture of the amniotic sac commonly occurs with effacement although it may happen later during labour;
    - amniotic fluid is released;
    - this is called spontaneous rupture of membranes.

MICRO-facts
When counselling a pregnant woman on how long labour will last:
- if it is their **first labour**: approx. 8–10 hours;
- if it is their **second labour**: approx. 6–8 hours.

- **Stages of labour**:
  - see Table 6.2.

Obstetrics

Table 6.2 Stages of labour.

	DEFINITION	PROCESSES	AVERAGE DURATION
First stage	Diagnosis of labour → full dilatation of the cervix (10 cm) **Latent phase:** 0–4 cm **Active phase:** 4–10 cm	**Latent phase:** Effacement Slow dilatation to 4 cm **Active phase:** Full dilatation at 1–2 cm/h **Movement of the head during the first stage** Engagement Descent Flexion Internal rotation	**Latent phase:** Very variable. May take many hours **Active phase:** Very variable. Roughly 2–6 hours. Depends on position
Second stage	Full dilatation → delivery of the fetus **Passive stage:** Fetal head is high; no maternal urge to push **Active stage:** Fetal head reaches pelvic floor. Active pushing occurs	Movement of the head: Completion of descent, flexion and internal rotation Extension Delivery	From the active stage: **Nulliparous:** 3 hours **Parous:** 2 hours
Third stage	Delivery of the fetus → delivery of the placenta	Uterus contracts and the placenta is delivered. Placental separation is marked by lengthening of the cord, a gush of blood per vaginum, and a hardening and rising of the uterus	15–30 minutes

Obstetrics

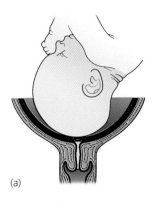

(a)

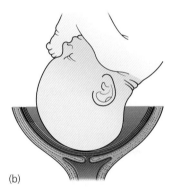

(b)

Fig. 6.3 (a) Uneffaced and (b) effaced cervix.

- **Mechanism of labour:**
  - The pelvic inlet is a different shape from the outlet.
  - The inlet is wider transversely, whereas the pelvic outlet is widest in the anterior–posterior diameter (see Fig. 6.4).
  - Consequently, the fetus changes position and attitude as it moves through the pelvis (see Fig. 6.5).
- **Station:**
  - descent of the head is measured on vaginal examination in relation to the ischial spines (see Fig. 6.6);
  - the level of descent is referred to as the **station**;
  - if the head is at the level of the ischial spines, the station = 0;
  - above the spines the station is negative (−3 to 0 cm);
  - below the spines the station is positive (0 to +3 cm).

Obstetrics

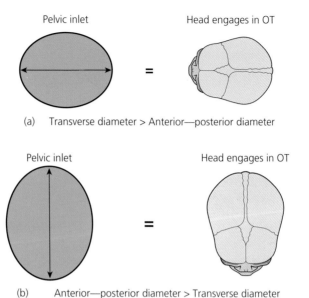

(a)   Transverse diameter > Anterior—posterior diameter

(b)   Anterior—posterior diameter > Transverse diameter

Fig. 6.4 **Pelvic dimensions and rotation of the head. OA, occiput anterior; OT, occiput transverse.**

6.3 MANAGEMENT OF NORMAL LABOUR

- **Introduction**:
  - Childbirth is a normal physiological process.
  - Thus, unnecessary clinical intervention should be minimized.

MICRO-reference

National Institute for Health and Clinical Excellence. Intrapartum care: care of healthy women and their babies during childbirth. NICE Clinical Guidance 55. London, UK: NICE, 2007. Available at http://www.nice.org.uk/nicemedia/pdf/IPCNICEGuidance.pdf

---

- **General principles**:
  - Support:
    - do not leave a labouring woman on her own;
    - the continuous presence of a birth partner shortens labour and reduces the need for pain relief and obstetric intervention.
  - Environment:
    - ideally, this should not be too clinical.
  - Encourage mobility.

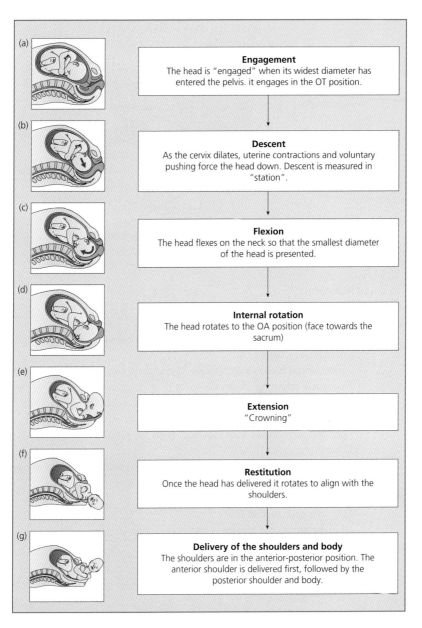

Fig. 6.5 (a–g) Movement of the head in labour. OA, occiput anterior; OT, occiput transverse.

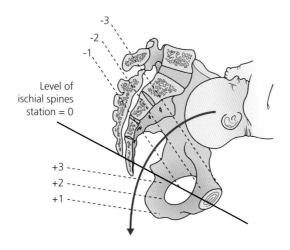

Fig. 6.6 **Level of descent (station).**

- Hydration:
  - encourage the woman to drink water.
- Nutrition:
  - a healthy woman with an uncomplicated pregnancy may eat a light diet during labour;
  - if the labour becomes complicated, general anaesthetic may be required;
  - stomach emptying slows down in pregnancy and labour;
  - the stomach contents can be aspirated (Mendelson's syndrome);
  - eating is contraindicated with opioid use or if the likelihood of general anaesthesia increases, e.g. poor progress.
- Micturition:
  - encourage the woman to urinate frequently to prevent detrusor damage;
  - monitor fluid balance.
- **Intra-partum care**:
  - With reference to Fig. 6.7:
    - For progress, the vaginal examination assesses:
      - ○ effacement;
      - ○ dilatation;
      - ○ station;
      - ○ position.

MICRO-print

Women should not deliver supine or semi-supine; in this position the gravid uterus may compress the abdominal aorta and inferior vena cava. This can lead to decreased cardiac output, hypotension and fetal distress. Skin-to-skin contact helps bonding and promotes oxytocin release.

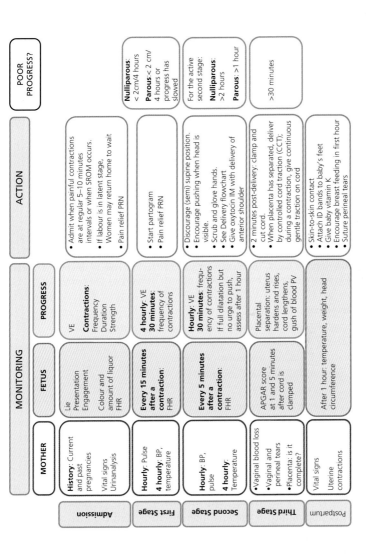

Fig. 6.7 Summary of intra-partum care. At each stage of labour, the mother, fetus and progress are monitored. The 'Action' column summarizes the necessary tasks for the stage of labour. The final column gives the definition for poor progress at each stage. BP, blood pressure; FHR, fetal heart rate; IM, intramuscularly; PRN, pro re nata; PV, per vaginum; SROM, spontaneous rupture of membranes; VE, vaginal examination.

Obstetrics

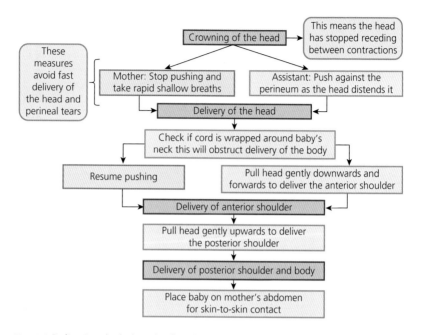

Fig. 6.8 Delivering the baby. This flowchart summarizes the role of the mother (green boxes) and assistant (orange boxes) during normal delivery of the baby.

- **The partogram**:
  - Graphic record of observations made in labour;
  - See Fig. 6.9.
  - Started from the diagnosis of labour.
  - Observations recorded include:
    - Progress:
      - cervical dilatation;
      - descent.
    - Maternal vital signs.
    - Fetal heart rate.
  - A '4 hour action line' is used to monitor progress:
    - This compares the rate of cervical dilatation during the active first stage with the average rate of 1 cm/h.
    - Dropping below the line indicates delay and requires attention.

MICRO-facts

Intramuscular oxytocin is given to the mother with the delivery of the anterior shoulder to stimulate placental separation. Once this has occurred, controlled cord traction is used to deliver the placenta. These measures shorten the third stage and reduce the risk of postpartum haemorrhage.

Obstetrics

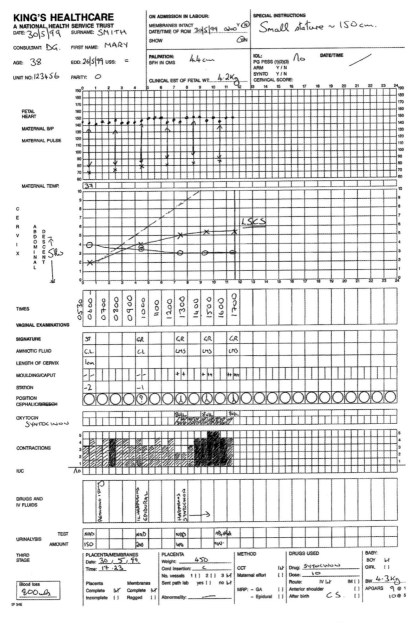

Fig. 6.9 The partogram. This is a partogram of a nulliparous woman of short stature with a big baby and an augmented labour. The labour culminates in an emergency caesarean section for cephalopelvic disproportion.

Obstetrics

- **Care of the neonate**:
  - APGAR score:
    - This is a tool used to describe the neonate's condition at birth.
    - It is recorded 1 minute and 5 minutes after the cord is clamped.
    - A low APGAR score prompts further monitoring or resuscitation.

Table 6.3 **APGAR score**.

	0	1	2
Appearance (trunk colour)	White/blue all over	Pink with blue extremities	Pink all over
Pulse rate	Absent	< 100 b.p.m.	> 100 b.p.m.
Grimace (response to stimulation)	Nil	Grimace	Cry/cough
Activity (tone)	Limp	Some flexion	Active, well-flexed movement
Respiratory effort	Absent	Gasping/irregular	Regular/strong cry

  - Vitamin K injection:
    - To prevent haemorrhagic disease of the newborn.

6.4 PAIN RELIEF

NON-PHARMACOLOGICAL

- **Transcutaneous electrical nerve stimulation (TENS)**:
  - **Procedure**:
    - Electrodes are placed on the woman's back.
    - Nerve fibres are stimulated with the aim of blocking pain impulses.
    - Advisable for the woman to practise before term.
  - TENS may be effective in early labour for some women.
  - There is no evidence to support its use in established labour.
- The following techniques may also help women to cope with labour pain:
  - breathing and relaxation: often the most effective;
  - hypnotherapy;
  - massage;
  - labouring in water;
  - acupuncture.

Obstetrics

> **MICRO-reference**
> National Institute for Health and Clinical Excellence. Intrapartum care:
> quick reference guide. NICE Clinical Guidance 55. London, UK: NICE,
> 2010. Available at http://guidance.nice.org.uk/CG55/QuickRefGuide/
> pdf/English.

INHALATIONAL ANALGESIA

- **Entonox**:
  - **Procedure**:
    - a combination of nitrous oxide and oxygen is inhaled through a mask or mouthpiece.
  - **Advantages**:
    - can be used throughout labour;
    - rapid onset;
    - does not cross the placenta; therefore, cannot affect the baby.
  - **Disadvantages**:
    - can cause nausea and light-headedness.

OPIATES

- **Pethidine and diamorphine**:
  - Intramuscular injection.
  - **Advantages**:
    - Can be patient controlled.
    - Easy administration.
    - Diamorphine is the best drug for primiparous women struggling with early labour.
  - **Disadvantages**:
    - Provides limited pain relief.
    - Significant side-effects including vomiting and drowsiness.
    - Can cause respiratory depression in the baby:
      - pethidine should not be given if delivery is expected within 2–3 hours. However, in the event that respiratory depression occurs it can be easily reversed using naloxone.

REGIONAL ANAESTHESIA

- **Spinal**:
  - **Procedure**:
    - injection of local anaesthetic into the cerebrospinal fluid (CSF).
  - **Advantages**:
    - effective analgesia;

- method of choice for caesarean section or mid-cavity instrumental vaginal delivery, if an epidural is not already *in situ*;
- relatively quick to administer.
- **Disadvantages**:
  - short-lasting;
  - complications include headache and total spinal block (hypotension, bradycardia, anxiety, apnoea and loss of consciousness); this is rare.
- See also Table 6.4 for advantages and disadvantages.
- **Pudendal block**:
  - lidocaine is injected around the pudendal nerve (sacral nerve roots 2, 3 and 4) bilaterally;
  - can be used for instrumental delivery.
- **Epidural**:
  - **Procedure**:
    - Injection of local anaesthetic into the epidural space (between the vertebrae L3 and L4).
    - Commenced once labour is established.
    - It can be infused continuously or with 'top-ups' approximately every 2 hours.
    - There is sensory (except pressure) and partial motor blockade from the upper abdomen downwards.
  - **Advantages**:
    - Most effective method of providing pain relief.
    - Fewer maternal and fetal risks than the use of systemic analgesia.
  - **Disadvantages**:
    - Side-effects:
      - loss of mobility;
      - postural hypotension.
  - See Table 6.4 for advantages and disadvantages:
    - Complications:
      - dural puncture: results in leakage of CSF and a severe headache;
      - injection of local anaesthetic into the CSF resulting in total spinal analgesia and respiratory paralysis;
      - bladder dysfunction can occur: the woman loses the urge to micturate and the bladder overfills, which can cause permanent damage to the detrusor muscle; if the woman is not voiding significant volumes spontaneously she should be catheterized.

> **MICRO-facts**
>
> Contraindications to epidural analgesia:
>
> - sepsis;
> - cardiovascular instability;
> - thrombocytopenia;
> - raised intra-cranial pressure;
> - unco-operative patient.

- **Combined spinal epidural anaesthesia:**
  - **Procedure:**
    - a large-bore needle is inserted into the epidural space and a fine-bore needle is inserted through this to puncture the subdural space.
  - **Advantages:**
    - quicker onset of pain relief than the use of epidural anaesthesia alone;
    - little or no motor blockade in most women;
    - patient-controlled dose.
  - **Disadvantages:**
    - see epidural anaesthesia above.

Table 6.4 Advantages and disadvantages of epidural versus spinal anaesthesia.

	EPIDURAL	SPINAL
Advantages	<ul><li>Most effective method of pain relief</li><li>Few maternal and fetal risks compared with systemic drugs</li></ul>	<ul><li>Effective</li><li>Method of choice for caesarean sections</li><li>Works more quickly</li><li>Segments are not missed</li></ul>
Disadvantages	<ul><li>Increased risk of instrumental delivery</li><li>Segment may be missed</li><li>Risk of dural puncture</li><li>Total spinal analgesia occurs if anaesthetic injected into the CSF (rare)</li><li>Risk of bladder dysfunction</li><li>Side-effects include loss of mobility and hypotension</li></ul>	<ul><li>Limited time span (2 hours)</li><li>Not suitable in woman with spina bifida or abnormal neurology</li><li>Headache</li><li>Risk of total spinal block</li><li>Hypotension: more common with a spinal than with an epidural</li></ul>

CSF, cerebrospinal fluid.

Obstetrics

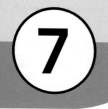

7 Complications in labour

7.1 POOR PROGRESS IN LABOUR

GENERAL PRINCIPLES

Three factors may result in poor progress. These are commonly referred to as 'the three Ps':

- **Powers**:
  - inefficient uterine action;
  - this is common in nulliparous women.
- **Passenger**:
  - Malpresentation:
    - Brow:
      - the width of this presenting part is incompatible with vaginal delivery, unless it converts to a face or vertex;
      - caesarean section is required.
    - Face:
      - if the chin is anterior (mento-anterior) vaginal delivery is possible;
      - if the chin is posterior (mento-posterior) vaginal delivery is not possible.
  - Malrotation:
    - Occiput posterior (OP):
      - the head is often extended in this position;
      - this presents a wider diameter;
      - OP may rotate to occiput anterior spontaneously;
      - if not, it may cause poor progress.
    - Occiput transverse (OT):
      - instrumental delivery may be necessary.
- **Passage**:
  - cephalo-pelvic disproportion: the maternal pelvis is too small or the fetus is too large; this is rarely the cause of poor progress;
  - resistance from the cervix and perineum.

MICRO-facts

If a multiparous woman has previously given birth by normal vaginal delivery, her poor progress is unlikely to be caused by inefficient uterine action. We also know that her pelvis is big enough unless this baby is particularly large. Therefore, malpresentation and malrotation are the most likely reasons for delay in multiparous women.

FIRST STAGE: POOR PROGRESS

- **Definition**:
  - nulliparous women: <2 cm cervical dilatation in 4 hours;
  - parous women: <2 cm cervical dilatation in 4 hours or a slowing in progress.
- **Assessment**:
  - To confirm delay in the first stage, the following are assessed:
    - rate of cervical dilatation;
    - uterine contractions: strength, frequency and duration;
    - presenting part: station and position;
    - how the woman is coping with the contractions and any pain;
    - fetal assessment (see 5.1 Fetal Monitoring in Chapter 5, Fetal growth and surveillance).
- **Management**:
  - Augmentation by amniotomy with/without intravenous oxytocin.
  - Amniotomy (artificial rupture of membranes (ARM)).
    - If spontaneous rupture of membranes has not occurred, this is done artificially.
    - It expedites labour and stimulates contractions.
  - Oxytocin.
    - If ARM has not been effective after 1–2 hours, intravenous oxytocin can be given.
    - It strengthens and increases the frequency of uterine contractions, thereby increasing cervical dilatation.
    - The woman should be offered an epidural before starting oxytocin.
    - Cardiotocography (CTG) must be used to monitor the fetus.
    - Complications:
      - ○ Uterine hyperstimulation. (1) Using too much oxytocin may cause excessively strong, frequent or prolonged contractions. (2) Because blood flow to the fetus is interrupted with each contraction, fetal distress can occur. (3) Management is with tocolytics, e.g. salbutamol, and caesarean section.
      - ○ Uterine rupture. (1) This is very rare in nulliparous women. (2) In multiparous women the risk is greater. (3) Malpresentation must be excluded before giving oxytocin.

Obstetrics

- Caesarean section:
  - if full dilatation does not occur after oxytocin.

SECOND STAGE: POOR PROGRESS

- **Definition**:
  - nulliparous women: active second stage >2 hours;
  - parous women: active second stage >1 hour.
- **Assessment**:
  - need for pain relief;
  - descent and position of fetus.
- **Management**:
  - Passive second stage:
    - intravenous oxytocin if descent is poor; delay pushing.
  - Active second stage:
    - if the fetal head is distending the perineum: episiotomy;
    - if the fetal head is too high: instrumental or operative delivery.

THIRD STAGE: POOR PROGRESS OR 'RETAINED PLACENTA'

- **Definition**:
  - For the actively managed third stage (i.e. oxytocin and controlled cord traction):
    - the placenta has not been delivered within 30 minutes of delivery of the baby.
- **Management**:
  - Oxytocin is injected into the umbilical vein and the cord is clamped proximally. This promotes placental separation.
  - If this fails, the placenta is removed manually under regional or general anaesthesia.
- **Complications**:
  - Postpartum haemorrhage (PPH):
    - the placenta may have partly separated from the uterus, causing significant haemorrhage.

MICRO-reference

National Institute for Health and Clinical Excellence. Intrapartum care: care of healthy women and their babies during childbirth. NICE Clinical Guidance 55. London, UK: NICE, 2007. Available at http://www.nice.org.uk/nicemedia/pdf/IPCNICEGuidance.pdf

---

Obstetrics

7.2 INDUCTION OF LABOUR

- **Definition**:
  - artificial initiation of labour.
- **Epidemiology**:
  - 1:5 deliveries are induced.
- **Indications**:
  - see Table 7.1.

MICRO-facts

Counselling the patient for induction:

- tell them that it is often more painful than spontaneous labour;
- discuss the options for pain control;
- the patient must be informed of the risk of possible caesarean section.

- **Procedure**:
  - The cervix is assessed by the Bishop's score to judge whether induction is likely to be successful:
    - This scoring system determines the favourability of the cervix; the lower the score the more likely induction is to fail.
  - **Cervical sweeping**:
    - This should be offered to women prior to formal induction.
    - In some cases it triggers spontaneous labour, preventing the need for induction.
    - A finger is passed through the cervix and a cyclical sweeping motion performed to separate the membrane surrounding the fetus from the cervix.

Table 7.1 Indications for induction of labour.

FETAL	MATERNAL	OBSTETRIC
Fetal growth restriction or compromise	Maternal disease, e.g. hypertension and diabetes	Pre-labour term rupture of membranes
	Social reasons	Prolonged pregnancy
		Pre-eclampsia
		Antepartum haemorrhage

Obstetrics

- **First-line – prostaglandins**:
  - Vaginal prostaglandins are the method of choice for the induction of labour.
  - They may be administered as a gel, tablet or pessary.
  - If there is deemed to be a risk of uterine hyperstimulation then an amniotomy with or without oxytocin should be considered instead.
- **Second-line – amniotomy and oxytocin**:
  - Amniotomy involves using an instrument called an amnihook to rupture the membranes.
  - An oxytocin infusion may be commenced following amniotomy if labour has not begun within 2 hours.
  - Provided the cervix is open and amniotomy is easy this is a suitable option.
- **Complications**:
  - Failure of induction resulting in caesarean section.
  - Uterine hyperstimulation:
    - this is rare but may result in fetal distress or uterine rupture.
  - Cord prolapse.
  - PPH.

MICRO-facts

Failed induction

- If this occurs the pregnancy and woman's condition should be reassessed.
- Further management options should be made in accordance with the mother's wishes.
- There are two options available:
  - a further attempt at induction;
  - caesarean section.

- **Contraindications to induction of labour**:
  - fetal compromise;
  - abnormal lie;
  - placenta praevia;
  - pelvic obstruction;
  - two previous caesarean sections.

MICRO-reference

National Institute for Health and Clinical Excellence. Induction of labour: full guideline. NICE Clinical Guidance 70. London, UK: NICE, 2008. Available at http://www.nice.org.uk/nicemedia/live/12012/41255/41255.pdf

7.3 PRE-TERM DELIVERY

- **Definition**:
  - delivery before 37 weeks' gestation.
- **Epidemiology**:
  - 8% of deliveries are pre-term;
  - the incidence has risen with assisted reproduction owing to an increase in multiple pregnancy.
- **Risk factors**:
  - Previous pre-term delivery:
    - this is the strongest predictor for recurrence.
  - Multiple pregnancies.
  - Sexually transmitted infections and ascent of commensal bacteria in the vagina through the cervix to the uterine cavity.
  - Fetal congenital or chromosomal abnormalities.
  - Social factors including:
    - increasing maternal age;
    - poverty;
    - alcohol and drug abuse.
  - Medical disorders including:
    - antepartum haemorrhage (APH);
    - pre-eclampsia.
  - Cervical incompetence:
    - associated with cervical trauma and infection.
- **Antenatal screening**:
  - Pre-term delivery is the most important cause of perinatal mortality.
  - Women with a history of the following are at high risk:
    - previous pre-term delivery;
    - recurrent cervical dilatation;
    - second trimester termination of pregnancy.
  - High-risk women may be screened for pre-term delivery by one of two methods:
    - measurement of fetal fibronectin;
    - measurement of cervical length.

MICRO-print
Fetal fibronectin

- Found in amniotic fluid and placenta.
- It is taken via a high vaginal swab in the late second or early third trimester.
- Its presence increases the risk of delivering before 34 weeks fourfold.
- If it is negative the woman is unlikely to go into labour within 14 days.

Obstetrics

> **MICRO-print**
> **Cervical length**
> - This is measured by transvaginal ultrasound scan.
> - It is usually only undertaken on women with a previous pre-term delivery.

- **Clinical features**:
  - History:
    - Abdominal pain.
    - Vaginal bleeding.
    - May be asymptomatic.
    - Presence of risk factors.
  - Examination:
    - Assess lie and presentation.
    - Are there regular contractions? This suggests labour has begun.
    - Speculum: assess degree of cervical effacement and dilatation:
      - ○ pre-term delivery may still occur even if the cervix is not dilating at the time of examination.
- **Investigations**:
  - Ultrasound:
    - cervical length (of little benefit in the acute situation);
    - fetal presentation;
    - placental position.
  - Fetal fibronectin (see above).
  - CTG:
    - to assess fetal well-being.
  - To identify infection:
    - high vaginal swab;
    - triple swabs;
    - urinalysis and mid-stream specimen of urine.

> **MICRO-facts**
> Pre-term labour is difficult to diagnose but identification of women at high risk can allow timely intervention.

- **Management**:
  - Steroids:
    - given between 24 and 34 weeks to reduce the severity of respiratory distress syndrome;
    - may take 48 hours to work.

- Tocolytics:
  - delay pre-term delivery;
  - often used in combination with steroids to allow time for them to have an optimal effect;
  - atosiban (oxytocin–vasopressin receptor blocker) and nifedipine (calcium channel blocker) are most commonly used.
- Antibiotics:
  - may be warranted if there is evidence of intra-uterine or extra-uterine infection.
- Mode of delivery:
  - vaginal delivery is the mode of choice;
  - most pre-term breeches will undergo a caesarean section;
  - caesarean section particularly at early gestation is associated with significant maternal morbidity.
- Delivery in pre-term labour is managed as a term delivery (see Chapter 6, Labour).

MICRO-facts

Ventouse delivery is contraindicated. Forceps may be used if indicated but they are not used routinely.

7.4 PRE-TERM/PRE-LABOUR RUPTURE OF MEMBRANES

- **Definition**:
  - rupture of membranes before labour and <37 weeks' gestation.
- **Epidemiology**:
  - occurs in 2% of pregnancies.
- **Aetiology**:
  - Risk factors:
    - Infection is the main cause:
      - bacterial vaginosis increases the risk of pre-term/pre-labour rupture of membranes (PPROM) 2.3-fold.
    - Placental abruption.
    - Polyhydramnios.
    - Multiple pregnancy.
    - Smoking.
    - Drug abuse.
- **Clinical features**:
  - History:
    - Gush of clear fluid vaginally.

- Examination:
  - If there is an infection, pyrexia and tachycardia will be present.
  - Abdomen:
    - ○ check lie and presentation;
    - ○ tenderness and 'woody' hardness suggests abruption;
    - ○ there may be contractions if labour has begun.
  - Speculum:
    - ○ usually performed after 40 minutes with the patient lying supine, to allow time for the liquor to collect.

MICRO-facts

Digital vaginal examination should not be performed as it increases the risk of infection.

- **Investigations**:
  - Urinalysis.
  - High vaginal swab.
  - Full blood count (FBC) and C-reactive protein.
  - Ultrasound:
    - to assess liquor volume and presentation.
  - CTG:
    - to assess fetal well-being.
- **Complications**:
  - pre-term delivery is the main complication;
  - infection;
  - cord prolapse (rare).
- **Management**:
  - The fundamental principle is to balance the risk of pre-term delivery against the risk of infection.
  - Delivery occurs spontaneously within 7 days in 80% of cases.
  - Corticosteroids are given.
  - Prevention of infection:
    - Prophylactic erythromycin should be given for 10 days following diagnosis.
    - The woman is monitored closely for signs of infection with 4 hourly temperature and pulse checks. The pulse rate may rise prior to the development of a pyrexia.
    - The baby is delivered if there are any signs of infection or fetal compromise.

- Delivery:
  - PPROM <24 weeks is associated with very poor survival rates for the baby and a discussion should be had with the parents. Some will consider termination.
  - If PPROM occurs between 24 and 34 weeks, expectant management should be attempted.
  - After 34 weeks' gestation, induction should be considered.

MICRO-facts

Chorioamnionitis

- **Definition**:
  - infection of the fetal membranes (amnion and chorion).
- **Aetiology**:
  - ascending infection from the vagina and cervix;
  - most commonly occurs after ruptured membranes and pre-term labour.
- **Symptoms**: include an offensive discharge and abdominal pain.
- **Management**:
  - if there is evidence of infection, broad-spectrum antibiotics should be given and delivery induced.

MICRO-reference

Royal College of Obstetricians and Gynaecologists. Preterm prelabour rupture of membranes. Green Top Guideline no. 44. London, UK: RCOG, 2006. Available at http://www.rcog.org.uk/files/rcog-corp/GTG44PPROM28022011.pdf

7.5 BREECH PRESENTATION

- **Definition**:
  - Presentation of the buttocks or feet.
  - Types of breech presentation (see Fig. 7.1):
    - extended (most common) – both knees are extended;
    - flexed – both knees are flexed;
    - footling – one or both feet present below the buttocks.
- **Epidemiology**:
  - at 28 weeks the incidence of breech presentation is about 20%;
  - this falls to 3% at term because most babies turn spontaneously;
  - affects 25% of pre-term births.

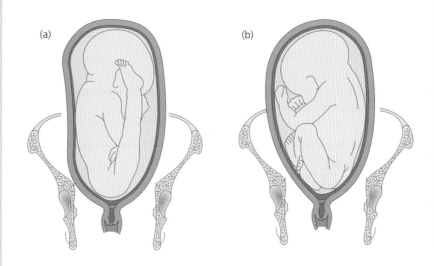

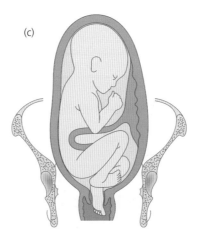

Fig. 7.1 Types of breech presentation. (a) Extension of the legs. (b) Flexion of the legs. (c) Footling.

- **Aetiology**:
  - majority of cases are idiopathic;
  - for the risk factors, see Table 7.2.
- **Clinical features**:
  - Breech presentation is commonly missed and often only detected at labour.
  - History:

Table 7.2 Risk factors for breech presentation and abnormal lie.

DECREASED UTERINE POLARITY	ALTERED FETAL MOBILITY	PREVENTION OF ENGAGEMENT
Multiparity	Fetal abnormality	Placenta praevia
Malformations	Prematurity	Pelvic tumour
	Multiple pregnancy	Uterine deformity
	Fetal growth restriction	

- – subcostal discomfort;
- – fetal movements felt predominantly in the lower abdomen.
  - Examination:
    - – palpable, ballotable head at fundus.
- **Investigations**:
  - Ultrasound:
    - – to confirm diagnosis and type of breech;
    - – to detect any contributing fetal or uterine abnormalities.
- **Complications**:
  - Increased perinatal mortality.
  - Fetal abnormalities.
  - Problems in labour:
    - – cord prolapse;
    - – trapping of the fetal head as it descends through the pelvis.

MICRO-facts

If the fetus's head is large or extended it may become trapped. Vaginal delivery is impossible. If the presentation is cephalic this is managed by caesarean section. In breech presentation it is too late for a caesarean section since the body has already been delivered. The baby will rapidly die.

- **Management**:
  - External cephalic version (ECV):
    - – May be performed after 37 weeks' gestation.
    - – Success rate is approximately 50%, which reduces the incidence of breech presentation at term to 1.5%.
    - – ECV best results are approximately 60–65% success.
    - – Procedure:
      - ○ performed under ultrasound guidance;
      - ○ both hands are placed on the mother's abdomen;

○ gentle pressure is applied in order to rotate the fetus, in the form of a somersault, into a vertex presentation;
○ facilities should be available for emergency caesarean section if complications arise;
○ anti-D is given to rhesus-negative women.
- Risks:
  ○ minimal;
  ○ placental abruption <1%;
  ○ prolonged fetal bradycardia;
  ○ pain.
- Contraindications:
  ○ compromised fetus;
  ○ placenta praevia;
  ○ multiple pregnancy;
  ○ ruptured membranes;
  ○ recent APH.

- Caesarean section:
  - This reduces the risk of perinatal and early neonatal mortality.
  - Following the Term Breech Trial, obstetric advice is that breech babies should be delivered by lower segment caesarean section (LSCS) because of reduced mortality and morbidity.
  - Some women will still request to have a vaginal breech birth; however, the number of people with the skills to deliver breech babies is dwindling.
- Vaginal breech birth:
  - The following factors are regarded as unfavourable for vaginal breech birth:
    ○ contraindications to vaginal birth (e.g. placenta praevia, compromised fetal condition);
    ○ clinically inadequate pelvis;
    ○ footling breech presentation;
    ○ large baby;
    ○ growth-restricted baby;
    ○ hyperextended fetal neck in labour.
  - Procedure:
    ○ the mechanism of labour is similar to a cephalic presentation;
    ○ an episiotomy is usually performed when the posterior buttock is delivering;
    ○ epidural analgesia is commonly used.

- Risks:
  - ○ incomplete cervical dilatation resulting in head entrapment;
  - ○ cord prolapse;
  - ○ traumatic injuries: (1) intra-cranial haemorrhage; (2) spinal cord damage; (3) nerve palsies.

MICRO-reference

Royal College of Obstetricians and Gynaecologists. The management of breech presentation. Green Top Guideline no. 20b. London, UK: RCOG, 2006. Available at http://www.rcog.org.uk/files/rcog-corp/GtG%20no% 2020b%20Breech%20presentation.pdf

---

7.6 ABNORMAL LIE (TRANSVERSE AND OBLIQUE)

- **Definition**:
  - transverse: the body lies across the uterus;
  - oblique: the head or buttocks are palpable in one iliac fossa.
- **Epidemiology**:
  - Affects 1:200 births.
  - More common in early pregnancy:
    - lie and presentation continually change >37 weeks' gestation.
- **Aetiology**:
  - Tends to affect pre-term births more commonly than term births.
  - Risk factors:
    - see Table 7.2.
- **Complications**:
  - Cannot deliver vaginally.
  - Arm or cord prolapse.
- **Clinical features**:
  - History:
    - the baby turns frequently.
  - Examination:
    - palpation of the fetal pole laterally (transverse lie) or in the right or left iliac fossa (oblique lie).
- **Investigations**:
  - ultrasound scan to confirm lie.

Obstetrics

- **Management**:
  - Common before 37 weeks – no action required.
  - If the fetal lie is abnormal after 37 weeks the following may be required:
    - Ultrasound scan to identify the cause.
    - Inpatient management: owing to the risk of cord prolapse if the membranes rupture:
      ○ if the baby spontaneously returns to and stays in a cephalic position for over 48 hours the woman can be discharged.
    - Caesarean section if the abnormal lie does not stabilize by 41 weeks.
    - Many women are reluctant to wait in hospital from 37 to 41 weeks and may push for an earlier LSCS.

7.7 ANTEPARTUM HAEMORRHAGE

- **Definition**:
  - vaginal bleeding between 24 weeks' gestation (the time of fetal viability) and the onset of delivery.
- **Causes**:
  - bleeding originates either from the placenta or from a local lesion in the cervix or vagina;
  - the local causes of APH are discussed in the relevant chapters.

Table 7.3 Causes of antepartum haemorrhage.

PLACENTAL	LOCAL
Placental abruption	Cervicitis
Placenta praevia	Cervical carcinoma
Vasa praevia	Vaginal infection/trauma

PLACENTAL ABRUPTION

- **Definition**:
  - separation of the placenta from the uterine wall.
- **Epidemiology**:
  - affects approximately 1% of pregnancies.
- **Risk factors**:
  - Intra-uterine growth restriction.
  - Pre-eclampsia.
  - Maternal smoking.
  - Previous history of placental abruption.

Obstetrics

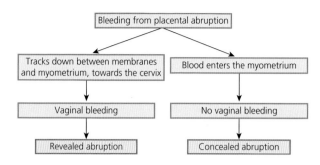

Fig. 7.2 Revealed and concealed abruptions.

- Uterine over-distension:
  - polyhydramnios;
  - multiple pregnancy.
- Hypertension.
- Trauma:
  - road traffic accidents;
  - external cephalic version (see Breech presentation).
- Maternal cocaine use (rare).
- **Pathophysiology (see Fig. 7.2)**:
  - As the placenta separates from the uterine wall, bleeding occurs.
  - If blood is passed vaginally it is a **revealed abruption**:
    - this accounts for two-thirds of abruptions.
  - Abruption may occur without subsequent vaginal bleeding. This is a **concealed abruption**:
    - this accounts for one-third of abruptions.
- **Clinical features**:
  - History:
    - Abdominal pain.
    - Vaginal bleeding:
      ○ often dark.

MICRO-facts

Remember that vaginal bleeding does **not** need to be present for placental abruption to be considered.

Also, tachycardia and hypotension which is out of proportion to any vaginal bleeding indicates that there may be an element of 'concealed' loss.

Obstetrics

- Examination:
  - Signs of shock.
  - Tender, hard uterus:
    - 'wooden'.
  - Diminished or absent fetal heart sounds.
- **Investigations**:
  - Clinical diagnosis.
  - Investigations are for monitoring maternal and fetal well-being.
  - Maternal:
    - Blood tests:
      - FBC;
      - cross-match;
      - coagulation screen;
      - urea and electrolytes.
    - Urinary catheterization:
      - to monitor urine output.
    - Ultrasound scan.
      - to exclude placenta praevia (see later).
  - Fetus:
    - CTG.

MICRO-facts

Any form of antepartum haemorrhage is a potential sensitizing event so rhesus-negative women must be given anti-D.

- **Management**:
  - admission;
  - intravenous fluids;
  - consider blood transfusion;
  - corticosteroids if <34 weeks' gestation;
  - opiate analgesia;
  - anti-D for rhesus-negative women.
- **Timing and mode of delivery**:
  - Depends on the presence or absence of the fetal heart rate.
  - Fetal heart rate (FHR) present:
    - fetal distress → urgent caesarean section;
    - if no fetal distress and ≥37 weeks → induction of labour;
    - if no fetal distress and <34 weeks → corticosteroids and monitor closely.
  - FHR absent:
    - vaginal delivery.

Obstetrics

- **Complications:**
  - see Table 7.4.

Table 7.4 Complications of placental abruption.

MATERNAL COMPLICATIONS	FETAL/NEONATAL COMPLICATIONS
Hypovolaemic shock	Intra-uterine growth restriction
Acute renal failure	Pre-term delivery
Disseminated intravascular coagulation	Stillbirth
Sensitization to rhesus D antigen	
Death	

- **Prognosis:**
  - high risk of developing PPH (see later).

PLACENTA PRAEVIA

- **Definition:**
  - the placenta occupies the lower segment of the uterus.
- **Classification:**
  - see Table 7.5.

Table 7.5 Definitions of placenta praevia.

MAJOR PRAEVIA	MINOR/PARTIAL PRAEVIA
The placenta covers the internal cervical os	The placenta occupies the lower uterine segment but does not cover the internal os

- **Epidemiology:**
  - Affects about 0.4% of pregnancies at term.
  - It is common for the placenta to be low lying at 20 weeks:
    - The lower segment of the uterus develops between 30 and 34 weeks' gestation. As a consequence, the majority of placentas that are low lying at 20 weeks appear to move up as the pregnancy progresses, when actually the uterus has developed below it.
  - Only 10% of 'low-lying' placentas will be praevia at term.
- **Risk factors:**
  - multiple pregnancy;
  - high parity;

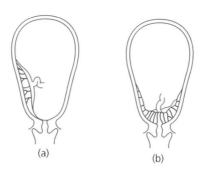

Fig. 7.3 Examples of (a) minor and (b) major placenta praevia.

- increased maternal age;
- previous caesarean section;
- uterine structural abnormality;
- assisted conception.
- **Clinical features**:
  - History:
    - **painless** vaginal bleeding.
  - Examination:
    - transverse lie;
    - high fetal head (as not engaged);
    - breech presentation.

> ## MICRO-facts
>
> Vaginal examination **should not** be carried out with antepartum haemorrhage; if there is placenta praevia it may provoke massive haemorrhage. However, if required, gentle speculum examination (with a Sims speculum) is acceptable.

- **Investigations**:
  - Diagnosis:
    - Abdominal ultrasound scan.
    - Transvaginal scan:
      ○ this is an ultrasound assessment of the distance between the leading placental edge and the internal os;
      ○ this is the gold standard for diagnosing placenta praevia.

- Maternal/fetal monitoring:
  - As for placental abruption.
- **Management**:
  - Admission:
    - if asymptomatic, admission can be delayed until 37 weeks.
  - May require blood transfusion.
  - Anti-D for rhesus-negative women.
  - Corticosteroids if <34 weeks' gestation.
- **Delivery**:
  - elective caesarean section at 39 weeks;
  - if there is severe bleeding → emergency caesarean section;
  - may consider vaginal delivery in some cases.
- **Complications**:
  - **Maternal**:
    - haemorrhage;
    - caesarean section;
    - placenta accreta;
    - placenta increta;
    - placenta percreta;
    - hysterectomy (due to massive haemorrhage).
  - **Fetal/neonatal**:
    - pre-term delivery.

MICRO-print
- Placenta accreta:
  - the placenta implants into the myometrium, commonly into a previous caesarean section scar;
  - it fails to separate from the myometrium after delivery.
- Placenta increta:
  - the placenta invades the myometrium.
- Placenta percreta:
  - the placenta invades through the entire uterine wall; it may implant into surrounding structures.

- **Prognosis**:
  - high risk of developing PPH as the lower uterine segment contracts poorly.

Table 7.6 Comparison of placental abruption and placenta praevia.

	PLACENTAL ABRUPTION	PLACENTA PRAEVIA
Pain	Yes, often severe	No
Bleeding	May or may not be present	Yes, often profuse
Shock	May be inconsistent with external loss	Usually consistent with external loss
Who is in most danger?	Fetus	Mother
Fetus	Normal lie and head engagement	Usually abnormal lie/head not engaged
Ultrasound	Often normal	Low-lying placenta

From Impey L, Child T. Obstetrics and gynaecology, 3rd edn. Oxford, UK: Wiley-Blackwell, 2008.

MICRO-print

Vasa praevia

- Defined as fetal blood vessels in the membranes covering the internal os and below the presenting part.
- Clinical features:
  - bleeding (fetal blood) from the vagina after amniotomy or spontaneous rupture of the membranes;
  - cardiotocography abnormalities.
- Fetal blood volume is only 80 mL/kg body weight so a swift loss may compromise the baby very quickly.
- Managed by urgent caesarean section.

MICRO-facts

Antepartum haemorrhage tends to weaken, but postpartum haemorrhage kills!

MICRO-reference

Royal College of Obstetricians and Gynaecologists. Placenta praevia, placenta praevia accreta and vasa praevia: diagnosis and management. Green Top Guideline no. 27. London, UK: RCOG, 2011. Available at http://www.rcog.org.uk/files/rcog-corp/GTG%2027%20Placenta%20Praevia%20January%202011.pdf

Obstetrics

7.8 POSTPARTUM HAEMORRHAGE

- **Definition**:
  - **Primary PPH**:
    - >500 mL blood loss in first 24 hours post-delivery.
  - **Secondary PPH**:
    - excessive blood loss from 24 hours up to 12 weeks post-delivery.
  - **Massive PPH**:
    - >1500 mL blood loss.
- **Causes**:
  - see Table 7.7.

Table 7.7 Causes of postpartum haemorrhage (PPH).

PRIMARY PPH	SECONDARY PPH
Atonic uterus	Endometritis
Perineal trauma	Retained products of conception
Vaginal/cervical tear	
Uterine rupture	

- **Risk factors**:
  - previous PPH;
  - APH;
  - coagulation abnormality;
  - retained placenta;
  - multiple pregnancy;
  - polyhydramnios;
  - prolonged labour (>12 hours);
  - induction of labour;
  - instrumental delivery;
  - caesarean section.

MICRO-facts

The causes of postpartum haemorrhage can be grouped into 'the four Ts':

- **T**one (abnormalities of uterine contraction).
- **T**issue (retained placental tissue).
- **T**rauma.
- **T**hrombin (clotting abnormalities).

Obstetrics

- **Prevention**:
  - prophylactic oxytocin is given to all women in the final stage of labour;
  - oxytocin causes uterine contraction;
  - this reduces PPH by 60%.
- **General management**:
  - Resuscitation:
    - Remember to assess patient using the ABCDE approach.
    - Oxygen.
    - Venous access with large-bore cannulae.
    - Commence intravenous fluids/blood transfusion with cross-matched blood.
  - Call for senior help.
  - Monitoring/investigations:
    - Blood tests:
      - cross-match;
      - FBC;
      - coagulation screen.
    - Monitor pulse, blood pressure and respiratory rate continuously.
    - Catheterize and monitor urine output.
  - Identifying cause:
    - Look for any genital tract trauma:
      - tears should be sutured in theatre with good lighting.
    - Treat the underlying cause.

ATONIC UTERUS

- **Definition**:
  - the uterus fails to contract after delivery.
- **Epidemiology**:
  - atonic uterus is the commonest cause of primary PPH.
- **Causes/risk factors**:
  - Over-distension of the uterus, e.g. with polyhydramnios.
  - Induction of labour:
    - this is evidence of insufficient uterine contraction.
  - Prolonged labour:
    - for example, as a result of malposition (occiput transverse or occiput posterior) (see Chapter 6, Labour);
    - the uterus tires, failing to contract.
- **Clinical features**:
  - Enlarged uterus:
    - around the level of umbilicus.
- **Specific management**:
  - Massage the uterus:
    - this stimulates uterine contraction.

- Catheterize and empty the bladder.
- Oxytocin, ergometrine and prostaglandins stimulate the uterus to contract.
- If these methods fail, an intra-uterine balloon tamponade, B-Lynch suture or hysterectomy may be used.
- **Complications**:
  - **Maternal**:
    - massive haemorrhage;
    - hysterectomy.

UTERINE RUPTURE

- **Epidemiology**:
  - 1:1500 pregnancies;
  - usually occurs during labour.
- **Risk factors**:
  - Scarred uterus:
    - classic caesarean scar (vertical incision) carries a higher risk than a lower segment scar;
    - myomectomy.
  - Congenital uterine abnormalities.
- **Clinical features**:
  - constant abdominal pain;
  - vaginal blood loss;
  - haematuria;
  - FHR abnormalities;
  - loss of contractions.
- **Specific management**:
  - Urgent laparotomy:
    - deliver fetus;
    - repair uterus/hysterectomy.
- **Complications**:
  - Maternal:
    - massive internal haemorrhage;
    - hysterectomy.
  - Fetal/neonatal:
    - hypoxia due to extrusion from the uterus.
- **Prognosis**:
  - high recurrence rate;
  - subsequent pregnancies should be managed with caesarean deliveries.

ENDOMETRITIS

- **Definition**:
  - infection confined to the uterus.
- **Risk factors**:
  - instrumental delivery;
  - caesarean section;
  - miscarriage;
  - termination of pregnancy;
  - retained products of conception.
- **Clinical features**:
  - abdominal/pelvic pain;
  - vaginal bleeding;
  - tender uterus;
  - fever and tachycardia;
  - cervical os often open.
- **Specific investigations**:
  - vaginal and cervical swabs;
  - pelvic ultrasound may help exclude retained products of conception.
- **Specific management**:
  - co-amoxiclav and metronidazole;
  - in severe cases, add in gentamicin;
  - may require evacuation of retained products of conception, especially if the cervical os is open.

RETAINED PRODUCTS OF CONCEPTION

- May or may not cause endometritis.
- **Specific management**:
  - Evacuation of retained products of conception:
    - under general anaesthesia;
    - cervix is dilated;
    - retained placental tissue is removed by a suction curette.

MICRO-reference

Royal College of Obstetricians and Gynaecologists. Prevention and management of postpartum haemorrhage. Green Top Guideline no. 52. London, UK: RCOG, 2009. Available at http://www.rcog.org.uk/files/rcog-corp/Green-top52PostpartumHaemorrhage.pdf

7.9 SHOULDER DYSTOCIA

- **Definition**:
  - dystocia means difficulty during labour;
  - in shoulder dystocia, the fetal shoulders become stuck behind the pubic symphysis after delivery of the head;
  - extra manoeuvres are required to deliver the fetal shoulders.
- **Epidemiology**:
  - affects around 1:200 deliveries.
- **Risk factors**:
  - Shoulder dystocia is unpredictable and unpreventable.
  - The following associated factors have been identified. However, they are poor predictors of shoulder dystocia, even if many are present:
    - previous shoulder dystocia;
    - macrosomia;
    - diabetes mellitus;
    - high maternal body mass index;
    - small mother;
    - assisted vaginal delivery;
    - prolonged first/second stage of labour.
- **Pathophysiology**:
  - the anterior shoulder may be stuck behind the maternal symphysis pubis;
  - the posterior shoulder may be impacted on the sacral bones.
- **Complications**:
  - **Maternal**:
    - vaginal tear;
    - primary postpartum haemorrhage;
    - emotional impact.
  - **Fetal/neonatal**:
    - cerebral damage;
    - brachial plexus injury;
    - shoulder/arm fracture;
    - death.

MICRO-facts

Brachial plexus injury

- This is caused by excessive traction at the neck.
- Usually temporary, but may be permanent.
- **Erb's palsy** can result.
  - Arm on the affected side is medially rotated and wrist is flexed.
  - Also known as the 'waiter's tip' sign.
- Can be a source for litigation.

Obstetrics

- **Management**:
  - Senior help.
  - McRoberts' manoeuvre:
    - mother's hips are hyperflexed and abducted;
    - suprapubic pressure may be added;
    - helpful in around 90% of cases.

MICRO-print

If the McRoberts' manoeuvre fails, the following may be considered:

- Wood's screw manoeuvre.
  - Pressure is applied behind the anterior shoulder and also the posterior shoulder.
  - Attempts are made to rotate the shoulders by this method.
- Symphysiotomy.
- Zavanelli manoeuvre:
  - Replacement of the head into the vagina followed by a caesarean section.

  - Good documentation:
    - helps protect against litigation;
    - it is also important to document which shoulder was anterior.
  - Good communication with the parents.
  - Debriefing with team.

MICRO-reference

Royal College of Obstetricians and Gynaecologists. Shoulder dystocia. Green Top Guideline no. 42. London, UK: RCOG, 2005. Available at http://www.rcog.org.uk/files/rcog-corp/uploaded-files/GT42ShoulderDystocia2005.pdf

---

7.10 UMBILICAL CORD PROLAPSE

- **Definition**:
  - The descent of the umbilical cord through the cervix after rupture of the membranes.
  - Occult cord prolapse (not visible on vaginal examination):
    - cord lies next to the presenting part.
  - Overt cord prolapse (visible on vaginal examination):
    - cord lies past the presenting part.
- **Epidemiology**:
  - affects around 1:500 deliveries.

- **Risk factors**:
  - Prematurity.
  - Breech presentation.
  - Polyhydramnios.
  - Unstable lie:
    - the lie of the fetus keeps changing.
  - Multiple pregnancy.
  - Artificial rupture of membranes.
- **Pathophysiology**:
  - The umbilical cord may be compressed between the presenting part and the pelvis or go into spasm (if its temperature is reduced), resulting in a reduced oxygen supply to the fetus.
- **Complications**:
  - **Fetal/neonatal**:
    - fetal hypoxia;
    - death.
- **Investigations**:
  - CTG:
    - may show abnormalities, e.g. bradycardia.
  - Vaginal examination:
    - may reveal cord prolapse.
- **Management**:
  - Avoid handling the cord as this may cause spasm.
  - The cord should remain in the vagina to keep it at body temperature.
  - If the cord is outside the body, it will cool and go into spasm.
  - Minimize cord compression by either manual elevation of the presenting part or filling the bladder, which will displace the presenting part.
  - Further reduce cord compression by encouraging the mother to adopt appropriate positions, e.g. knee–chest position.
  - Caesarean section is usually recommended (unless delivery is imminent).
  - Vaginal delivery may be considered if the cervix is fully dilated.
- **Prognosis**:
  - depends upon many factors, such as gestation and duration of cord compression;
  - prognosis is excellent for term babies if diagnosed early and in hospital.

MICRO-reference

Royal College of Obstetricians and Gynaecologists. Umbilical cord prolapse. Green Top Guideline no. 50. London, UK: RCOG, 2008. Available at http://www.rcog.org.uk/files/rcog-corp/uploaded-files/ GT50UmbilicalCordProlapse2008.pdf

Obstetrics

7.11 AMNIOTIC FLUID EMBOLISM

- **Definition**:
  - amniotic fluid entering the maternal circulation, causing cardiorespiratory compromise.
- **Epidemiology**:
  - very rare;
  - affects around 1:50 000 pregnancies.
- **Risk factors**:
  - strong uterine contractions in the presence of polyhydramnios.
- **Pathophysiology**:
  - the exact mechanism is unknown.
- **Clinical features**:
  - **Symptoms**:
    - sudden, severe chest pain;
    - shortness of breath.

> **MICRO-print**
> An amniotic fluid embolus is usually a post-mortem diagnosis.

- **Signs**:
  - Hypotension.
  - Tachycardia.
  - Hypoxia:
    ○ may lead to seizures.
  - Pulmonary oedema.
  - Haemorrhage:
    ○ due to disseminated intravascular coagulation.
- **Investigations**:
  - FBC.
  - Urea and electrolytes.
  - Cross-match.
  - Coagulation screen.
  - ECG:
    - may show right ventricular strain.
  - Arterial blood gas:
    - will show hypoxia.
- **Management**:
  - resuscitation and circulatory support;
  - oxygen therapy (intubation may also be needed);
  - cross-matched blood and fresh frozen plasma (contains clotting factors);
  - transfer to intensive treatment unit.

- **Prognosis**:
  - 80% maternal mortality rate.

7.12 UTERINE INVERSION

- **Definition**:
  - Inversion of the uterine fundus into the uterine cavity:
    - it may descend through the cervix or the vulva.

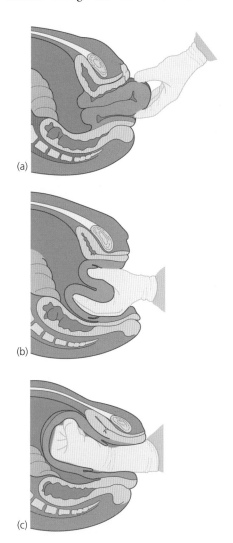

(a)

(b)

(c)

Fig. 7.4 (a) Example of uterine inversion; (b–c) manual replacement of the uterus.

- **Epidemiology**:
  - very rare;
  - 1:20 000 deliveries affected.
- **Risk factors**:
  - traction on the placenta.
- **Clinical features**:
  - haemorrhage;
  - pain;
  - hypotension.
- **Management**:
  - Immediate manual replacement of the uterus through the cervix (see Fig. 7.4. (b–c)).
  - If this fails, a general anaesthetic is given and the uterus is replaced with hydrostatic pressure using warm saline.
  - Do not remove the placenta until the normal anatomy is achieved.

8 Obstetric procedures

8.1 PERINEAL CARE

PERINEAL TEARS

- **Definition**:
  - any trauma to the perineum during childbirth.
- **Classification**:
  - see Table 8.1.

Table 8.1 Classification of perineal tears.

DEGREE	FEATURES
First	Only skin involved
Second	Perineal muscle involvement (includes all episiotomies)
Third	Second degree tear + involvement of anal sphincter
Fourth	Third degree tear + involvement of anal epithelium

- **Epidemiology**:
  - can occur in up to 70% of deliveries.
- **Management**:
  - should be sutured appropriately;
  - local or generalized anaesthesia may be required;
  - some first degree tears may not need to be sutured;
  - third degree tears and above need to be sutured in theatre.
- **Complications**:
  - haemorrhage;
  - haematoma;
  - fistula;
  - superficial dyspareunia;

- scarring;
- infection;
- faecal incontinence (for third/fourth degree tears).

MICRO-reference

Royal College of Obstetricians and Gynaecologists. The management of third- and fourth- degree perineal tears. Green Top Guideline no. 29. London, UK: RCOG, 2007. Available at http://www.rcog.org.uk/files/rcog-corp/uploaded-files/GT29ManagementThirdFourthDegreeTears2007.pdf

---

EPISIOTOMY

- **Definition**:
  - a surgical incision made in the perineum during delivery to widen the vulval outlet and reduce the risk of natural perineal tearing.

MICRO-facts

Natural perineal tears may be extensive and harder to repair than episiotomies.

- **Epidemiology**:
  - in England (2002–3), 13% of pregnant women had an episiotomy.
- **Indications**:
  - fetal distress;
  - shoulder dystocia;
  - instrumental delivery;
  - inelastic perineum;
  - fetal malposition.
- **Technique**:
  - A sharp, straight pair of scissors is used to make a single cut.
  - **Mediolateral episiotomy**:
    - commonly used in the UK;
    - cut starts in the midline and is then directed diagonally to avoid the anal sphincter.
  - **Midline episiotomy**.
    - uncommon in the UK;
    - still used in the USA;
    - cut starts in the midline and is directed towards the anus;
    - there is a risk of third/fourth degree perineal tears (see Table 8.1).

- **Repair**:
  - as per management of perineal tears.
- **Complications**:
  - as per complications of perineal tears.

8.2 INSTRUMENTAL DELIVERIES

- **Definition**:
  - the use of forceps or a ventouse to assist in delivering a baby vaginally.

Table 8.2 **Types of instruments.**

INSTRUMENT	DESCRIPTION
Forceps	A pair of blades that fits around the fetal head. Can be **non-rotational,** allowing traction only, or **rotational,** allowing the head to be rotated as well as traction
Ventouse	A metal or rubber cap that is connected to a vacuum pump. The cap is applied to the fetal head

- **Indications**:
  - Inadequate progress of second stage of labour:
    - >3 hours for nulliparous women;
    - >2 hours for multiparous women.
  - Maternal exhaustion during the second stage of labour.
  - Fetal distress during the second stage of labour.
  - To assist delivering the head after breech delivered vaginally.
  - Reducing the effect of the second stage of labour on medical conditions:
    - cardiac disease;
    - hypertension.
- **Conditions for an instrumental delivery**:
  - The following conditions should be met before considering an instrumental delivery:
    - The head should be at or below the level of the ischial spines on vaginal examination.
    - The fetal head should not be palpable abdominally.
    - The cervix should be fully dilated.
    - The position of the fetal head is known.

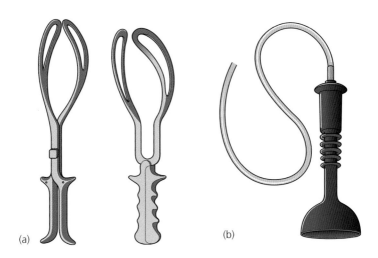

(a)   (b)

Fig. 8.1 (a) Forceps and (b) ventouse instruments.

- – Adequate analgesia is given.
- – The bladder is emptied, usually by catheterization.
- – Consent:
  - ○ this can be verbal;
  - ○ it is good practice to document what has been discussed and that consent has been obtained.
- – A skilled operator is available to perform or supervise the delivery.
- **Forceps or ventouse?**
  - Ventouse delivery is contraindicated for:
    - – face presentation;
    - – gestation <34 weeks;
    - – active bleeding from a fetal scalp blood sampling site.
  - In these scenarios, forceps should be used.
- **Complications**:
  - see Tables 8.3 and 8.4.

> **MICRO-reference**
> Royal College of Obstetricians and Gynaecologists. Operative vaginal delivery. Green Top Guideline no. 26. London, UK: NICE, 2011. Available at http://www.rcog.org.uk/files/rcog-corp/GTG26.pdf

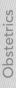

Obstetrics

Table 8.3 Complications of forceps delivery.

MATERNAL	FETAL
Uterine trauma	Facial bruising
Cervical trauma	Facial nerve injury
Vaginal trauma	Skull fractures
Perineal tears	Neck fractures
Haemorrhage	

Table 8.4 Complications of ventouse delivery.

MATERNAL	FETAL
Vaginal trauma	'Chignon' (swollen area of scalp where the cup was attached)
Perineal tears	Scalp lacerations
Haemorrhage	Neonatal jaundice
	Cephalhaematomata (subperiosteal haemorrhage)

8.3 CAESAREAN SECTION

- **Definition**:
  - An operation that allows a baby to be delivered via the abdomen.
  - **Emergency caesarean section**:
    - performed during labour;
    - usually done because of immediate threat to the mother or fetus.
  - **Elective caesarean section**:
    - planned at a time to suit the mother and to avoid labour;
    - performed at 39 weeks' gestation.
- **Epidemiology**:
  - in England (2002–3), the lower segment caesarean section (LSCS) rate was around 22%.
- **Indications**:
  - see Table 8.5.
- **Technique**:
  - **LSCS**:
    - a suprapubic transverse incision is made in the abdominal wall;
    - the lower segment of the uterus is then incised transversely and the baby is delivered;

Obstetrics

Table 8.5 Indications for elective and emergency caesarean sections.

ELECTIVE CAESAREAN SECTION	EMERGENCY CAESAREAN SECTION
Placenta praevia	Poor progress in labour
Non-correctable fetal lie	Fetal distress
Breech presentation	
Previous caesarean section	
Maternal medical problems that require a controlled delivery	

- the placenta is delivered by continuous cord traction;
- the uterus and abdominal wall are sutured in layers.
  - **Classic caesarean section**:
    - rare;
    - usually done when there is no lower segment, i.e. with very premature babies;
    - same as a LSCS, except vertical incisions are used.
- **Complications**:
  - Maternal haemorrhage.
  - Infection of the uterus or wound:
    - minimized with prophylactic antibiotics.
  - Maternal bladder/bowel damage.
  - Maternal venous thromboembolism.
  - Complications with anaesthesia.
  - Fetal lacerations.
  - Risk of uterine rupture during labour in subsequent pregnancies.

MICRO-facts

Caesarean sections increase the risk of placenta praevia in subsequent pregnancies. This is because the placenta is more likely to implant onto the scar of a lower segment caesarean section.

For more information on placenta praevia, see Chapter 7, Complications in labour.

MICRO-print
Maternal requests for elective caesarean sections are becoming more common. This may be due to anxieties regarding natural childbirth. If this is the case, the woman should be provided with perinatal mental health support. If vaginal birth is still unacceptable, then a planned caesarean section should be offered.

9 Puerperium

9.1 INTRODUCTION

- The puerperium is the 6 week period following delivery of the baby.
- During this period the body returns to its pre-pregnancy state physiologically.
- There is little obstetric input during this time yet it is the period associated with the greatest maternal morbidity and mortality.

PHYSIOLOGICAL CHANGES

- These are described in Fig. 9.1.

> **MICRO-facts**
>
> **Lochia**
>
> This is the discharge from the uterus. For the first 3 days it is red, then yellow, then white for the next 10 days. It is usually present for up to 6 weeks.

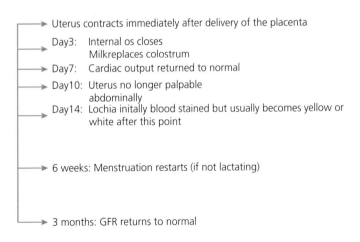

Fig. 9.1 **Time-line of physiological changes during the puerperium.**

GENERAL POST-NATAL CARE

- **Pre-discharge**:
  - Monitor fluid balance to prevent urinary retention.
  - Encourage early mobilization.
  - Give information and guidance on breast-feeding.
  - Teach pelvic floor exercises.
  - The following are checked daily:
    - temperature;
    - blood pressure;
    - perineal wounds;
    - lochia: persistent red lochia suggests retained products;
    - fundal height.
  - Anti-D should be given to rhesus-negative women within 72 hours of delivery.
  - Some women may wish to be discharged within 6 hours of delivery; this is the minimum recommended time, but others may need to stay in for longer.
- **Post-discharge**:
  - Rubella vaccination if non-immune, but if anti-D has been given then delay until post-natal examination.
  - The community midwife will visit, in some cases daily, for 10 days following discharge.
  - Contraception should be started within 3 weeks of delivery:
    - lactation suppresses ovulation but is not adequate contraception.
  - The 6–8 week post-natal examination is useful to assess maternal physical and mental well-being.

9.2 MEDICAL PROBLEMS

POSTPARTUM HAEMORRHAGE

- See Chapter 7, Complications in labour.

PUERPERAL PYREXIA

- **Definition**:
  - temperature $>38°C$ in the first 14 days.
- **Aetiology**:
  - urinary and genital tract infection account for the majority of cases;
  - most commonly occurs following caesarean section.
- **Examination**:
  - It is important to fully examine chest, breasts, legs, lochia, any wounds and perform a bimanual examination in order to try and identify a source of infection.

Obstetrics

- **Investigations**:
  - blood, urine, sputum and high vaginal cultures.
- **Treatment**:
  - broad-spectrum antibiotics.

PRE-ECLAMPSIA AND ECLAMPSIA

- Can start anew in the post-natal period (for clinical features, diagnosis and treatment, see Chapter 3, Medical problems in pregnancy).
- Within the first 72 hours after birth, women should be advised to seek immediate healthcare if they develop a headache plus at least one of:
  - visual disturbances;
  - nausea;
  - vomiting.
- Requires careful monitoring and treatment with anti-hypertensives.
- This may take up to 24 hours to resolve following delivery of the baby and in some cases much longer.

VENOUS THROMBOEMBOLISM

- This may present as deep vein thrombosis (DVT) or pulmonary embolism (PE).
- Pregnancy and the puerperium is a hypercoagulable state; therefore, it is very important to monitor for symptoms and signs of venous thromboembolism (VTE) in the antenatal, intra-partum and postpartum periods.
- Need for thromboprophylaxis should be considered and reviewed pre-booking, throughout the antenatal period, if admitted to hospital, intra-partum and postpartum.
- **Epidemiology**:
  - risk of VTE is highest in the post-natal period. It is the leading cause of maternal mortality.
- **Clinical features**:
  - DVT: unilateral calf pain, swelling or redness;
  - pulmonary embolism: shortness of breath or chest pain;
  - clinical signs may be absent in both cases.
- **Investigations**:
  - ECG: sinus tachycardia;
  - D-dimer will be raised; however, it is often raised in pregnancy;
  - arterial blood gas: a PE may cause hypoxia (low PaO_2);
  - Doppler: to exclude a DVT;
  - computed tomography pulmonary angiogram: if there is a high index of suspicion of PE.
- **Management**:
  - early mobilization is encouraged in order to reduce the risk of VTE;
  - low-molecular-weight heparin is commenced if there is a strong clinical suspicion of DVT/PE;

- once a DVT or PE is confirmed the woman can be started on warfarin, provided she consents;
- anti-coagulant treatment is usually 6 weeks for a DVT and 3 months for a PE.

MENTAL HEALTH

- **Post-natal blues**:
  - **Definition**:
    - transient low mood.
  - **Epidemiology**:
    - common post-natally;
    - tends to peak at day 4–5.
  - **Management**:
    - women should be given support and reassurance.
- **Post-natal depression**:
  - **Definition**:
    - depression that occurs within 4 weeks of childbirth.
  - **Epidemiology**:
    - the prevalence is between 4.5% and 28%.
  - **Management**:
    - social support and psychotherapy;
    - anti-depressants may be required.
- **Puerperal psychosis**:
  - **Definition**:
    - sudden onset of psychotic symptoms including hallucinations, mania, depression and a suicidal drive.
  - **Epidemiology**:
    - affects 0.1–0.2% women;
    - the suicide rate is 5% and the infanticide rate is 4%.
  - **Management**:
    - first, an organic cause of the psychosis is excluded;
    - requires psychiatric admission, ideally to a mother and baby unit under the supervision of a perinatal mental health team.

URINARY TRACT PROBLEMS

- **Urinary retention**:
  - **Definition**:
    - painful inability to void (note: there may not be any pain following an epidural);
    - common following delivery.

Obstetrics

- Management:
  - fluid balance should be monitored;
  - ensure the bladder does not get overdistended;
  - if the woman does not pass urine within 6 hours after the birth, the bladder volume should be assessed and catheterization considered.
- **Urinary incontinence**:
  - **Definitions**:
    - see Chapter 15, Urogynaecology.
  - **Epidemiology**:
    - affects 20% of women.
  - **Management**:
    - women should be taught pelvic floor exercises, which should be continued life-long after a vaginal birth;
    - if symptoms do not resolve, it will require further assessment.

BOWEL PROBLEMS

- **Constipation**:
  - give dietary advice;
  - laxatives may be required.
- **Faecal incontinence**:
  - **Epidemiology**:
    - affects approximately 4% of women.
  - **Aetiology**:
    - usually results from anal sphincter or pudendal nerve damage.
  - **Risk factors include**:
    - forceps delivery and shoulder dystocia.
  - **Management**:
    - physiotherapy with/without sphincter repair is the mainstay of treatment.

PERINEAL TRAUMA

- **Epidemiology**:
  - up to 85% of women experience some perineal trauma during vaginal birth;
  - perineal pain affects up to 80% of women in the first days post-natally and many still have discomfort at day 10.
- **Management**:
  - tears are repaired following delivery of the placenta;
  - topical cold therapy, e.g. crushed ice or gel pads, may provide some relief when applied to the perineal area.

- **Complications**:
    - superficial dyspareunia is common and may be eased with lubricant gel.

MICRO-reference

National Institute for Health and Clinical Excellence. Routine postnatal care of women and their babies. London, UK: NICE, 2006. Available at http://www.nice.org.uk/nicemedia/live/10988/30144/30144.pdf

---

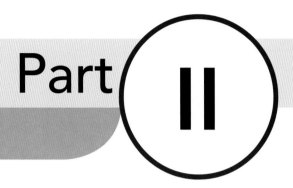

Part II

Gynaecology

10 Gynaecology: history and examination

10.1 HISTORY

The following should be included in addition to the standard medical history. For more detail for each section, please also see the relevant chapters.

MENSTRUAL HISTORY

- Age of first menstruation (menarche).
- Last menstrual period:
    - recorded as the first day of the last period.
- Menstrual cycle.

> **MICRO-facts**
>
> The menstrual cycle is usually expressed as X/Y.
>
> - Duration (X): for how many days does menstruation last?
> - Cycle (Y): how often does menstruation occur? (Number of days from first day of bleeding until the next first day.)
> - For example, 7/28 means menstruation lasts for 7 days and occurs every 28 days.

- Regular or irregular.
- Establish amount of bleeding:
    - number of pads/tampons used per day;
    - how often pads/tampons are changed;
    - clots/flooding (both indicate heavy bleeding);
    - impact on life.
- Non-menstrual bleeding:
    - inter-menstrual bleeding;
    - post-coital bleeding;
    - post-menopausal bleeding.
- Pain.
- Vaginal discharge.
- Age of menopause.

BRIEF PAST OBSTETRIC HISTORY

See also Chapter 1, Obstetrics: history and examination.
- Gravidity.
- Parity.
- Any complications with previous pregnancies or deliveries?

URINARY/PROLAPSE SYMPTOMS

- Urinary frequency.
- Nocturia.
- Urinary urgency.
- Urinary incontinence.
- Dragging sensation in vagina.
- Lump or mass in vagina.

SEXUAL/CONTRACEPTION HISTORY

- It is important to consider a genital tract infection when taking a gynaecological history (depending on the age of the patient).
- Pain during intercourse (dyspareunia).
- What form of contraception is used currently?
- What contraception has been used previously?

MICRO-facts

This may not always be appropriate, but bear in mind the possibility of domestic violence. Unfortunately, it still occurs quite commonly.

For more information see http://www.womensaid.org.uk/

CERVICAL SMEAR HISTORY (IF OVER 25 YEARS OLD)

- When was this last done?
- Any abnormal smears?
    - if so, what was done about them?

PAST MEDICAL HISTORY

- Gynaecological operations.
- Thyroid problems.

DRUG HISTORY

- If post-menopausal, is the patient on hormone replacement therapy?

FAMILY HISTORY

- Breast cancer.
- Gynaecological cancer.

10.2 EXAMINATION

GENERAL EXAMINATION

- Check for signs of anaemia:
  - pale conjunctiva;
  - pale palmar creases;
  - facial pallor.
- Assess pulse:
  - may help highlight underlying disease, e.g. thyroid disease;
  - tachycardia with a low blood pressure may suggest acute blood loss.
- Measure the patient's blood pressure.
- Check her body mass index.

MICRO-facts

Body mass index = Weight in kilograms (kg)/Height in metres $(m)^2$

ABDOMINAL EXAMINATION

In addition to a standard abdominal examination:

- Inspect for:
  - Scars from gynaecological/obstetric operations:
    - laparoscopic scars;
    - lower segment caesarean scars.
  - Distribution and quantity of body hair.
- Palpation:
  - Palpate for masses from above the umbilicus towards the symphysis pubis.
  - If there is a mass, can you get below it?
    - if not, the mass arises from the pelvis.

VAGINAL EXAMINATION

- Important points to remember:
  - ensure adequate privacy;
  - explain what you will be doing and obtain consent;
  - allow the patient to use the bathroom beforehand;
  - use gloves and lubricating gel for fingers and instruments;

Gynaecology

- metal instruments should be warmed before use;
- ensure there is a good, moveable light.

MICRO-facts

As this is an intimate examination, **always** ensure that a chaperone is present!

- Inspection:
  - Part the labia with your forefinger and thumb.
  - Are there any colour changes?
    - purple lesions → lichen planus;
    - pink–white lesions → lichen sclerosus.
  - Are there any ulcers or lumps on the vulva?
  - Ask the patient to strain. Is there any evidence of a prolapse (see Chapter 15, Urogynaecology)?
  - Ask the patient to cough. Is there leakage of urine (see Chapter 15, Urogynaecology)?
- Digital bimanual examination:
  - The patient should lie on her back with her legs flexed at the hip and the knee. Ask her to bring her heels together and up to her bottom, allowing her knees to fall down to the sides (abduction of knees).
  - Warn the patient when you are about to start the examination.
  - Place your left hand on the abdomen above the symphysis pubis.
    - This hand should be pushed down when trying to palpate the pelvic organs.
  - Insert your right index finger ($\pm$ right middle finger) into the vagina and feel for the following:
    - **Cervix:**
      - ○ Described as feeling like the 'tip of the nose' when non-pregnant and like 'lips' when pregnant.
      - ○ Is it irregular?
      - ○ Try to move the cervix. Does it cause any tenderness (cervical excitation)? Cervical excitation could be a sign of peritoneal irritation due to infection or bleeding.
    - **Uterus:**
      - ○ With your left hand pushing down on the abdomen, push the cervix upwards with your fingers (see Fig. 10.1).
      - ○ You should be able to feel the fundus of the uterus tapping your left hand.
      - ○ Assess: (1) size; (2) shape; (3) regularity; (4) tenderness; and (5) position. Anteversion: the uterus can be palpated by the

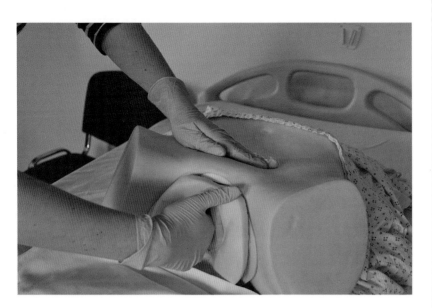

Fig. 10.1 Palpating the uterus.

method described above. Retroversion: the uterus cannot be palpated by the method mentioned above. If the uterus is retroverted, the cervix is very anterior, just behind the symphysis.
- **Adnexae (lateral fornices)**:
  ○ These are the spaces on either side of the uterus that contain the fallopian tube and ovary.
  ○ With your left hand pushing down on the abdomen, explore the adnexae.
  ○ Assess: (1) mass?; (2) tenderness? The ovaries and fallopian tubes are not usually palpable unless the woman is very thin.
- **Posterior fornix**:
  ○ Place your fingers behind the cervix.
  ○ The uterosacral ligaments can sometimes be palpated, e.g. nodules of endometriosis.
● **Bivalve (Cusco's) speculum examination** (see Figs. 10.2–10.6).
  ● Used to visualize the cervix and vaginal walls.
  ● Triple swabs or cervical smears can be done during this examination.
  ● Before removal, loosen the screw on the speculum and allow it to close as you withdraw it from the vagina.
  ● Prevent the speculum from catching on removal and inspect the vaginal walls to check for any abnormalities (bleeding, discharge, trauma).

Gynaecology

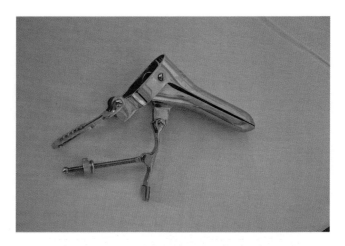

Fig. 10.2 Metal Cusco's speculum. These can also be plastic. Metal speculums can be sterilized and reused. Plastic ones are disposable.

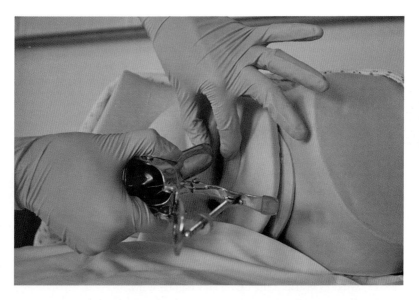

Fig. 10.3 Initial approach. The labia should be parted and the speculum held and inserted in the position shown.

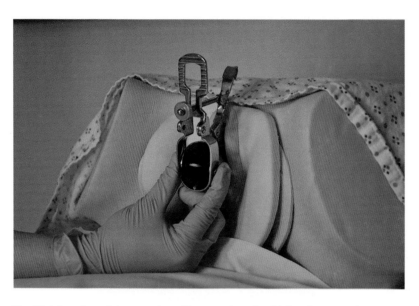

Fig. 10.4 Rotation of the speculum. The speculum should then be rotated anti-clockwise by 90°.

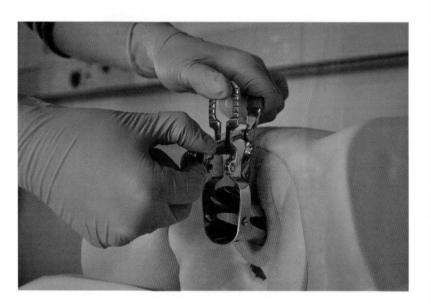

Fig. 10.5 Opening the speculum. Gently part the speculum and turn the screw to keep it fixed open.

Gynaecology

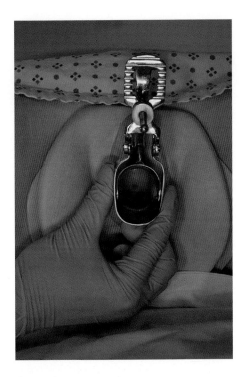

Fig. 10.6 **Visualize the cervix.**

- **Sim's speculum examination** (see Fig. 10.7).
  - This is for examining prolapses and vaginal walls.
  - The patient should be in the left lateral position, with her right leg flexed at the hip and knee and brought up to the abdomen. The left leg should be extended.
  - Place the speculum against the anterior or posterior vaginal wall. While the patient strains down, inspect the opposite wall for prolapse.

RECTAL EXAMINATION

- May be useful in differentiating between an enterocele and a rectocele.
- This may be useful in differentiating between per vaginal and per rectal bleeding.
- Also needed for excluding vault recurrence from cancer:
  - one finger is placed in the vagina and one in the rectum, simultaneously.

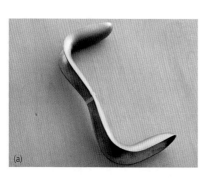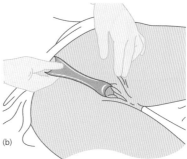

Fig. 10.7 (a) A Sim's speculum (b) examination with a Sim's speculum for anterior wall vaginal prolapse.

MICRO-facts

After a vaginal and/or a rectal examination, you must remember to record the following in the patient's notes:

- date;
- time;
- verbal consent obtained;
- name of the chaperone;
- grade of the chaperone, e.g. healthcare assistant, staff nurse;
- examination findings.

Reproductive endocrinology

11.1 THE NORMAL MENSTRUAL CYCLE

The changes in hormone levels during the menstrual cycle affect both the ovaries and the endometrium. The following is a simplified account of the normal menstrual cycle.

- **Days 1–4: menstruation**:
  - The endometrium is shed owing to a lack of hormonal support.
- **Days 5–13: proliferative/follicular phase**:
  - Gonadotrophin-releasing hormone from the hypothalamus stimulates release of follicle-stimulating hormone (FSH) and luteinizing hormone (LH) from the pituitary gland.
  - This happens because there is a lack of oestrogen, so there is little negative feedback on the hypothalamic–pituitary–ovarian (HPO) axis (see Fig. 11.1).
  - Multiple follicles are stimulated to grow and start producing oestrogen.
  - One follicle becomes 'dominant' and secretes a large amount of oestrogen.
  - This exerts a strong negative feedback on the HPO axis and reduces FSH secretion.
  - This causes atresia of the non-dominant follicles.
  - The oestrogen level continues to rise and reaches a point where it starts exerting a positive feedback effect on the HPO axis.
  - The oestrogen has a proliferative effect on the endometrium and causes it to thicken.
  - The increasing oestrogen level causes a LH surge (usually around 36 hours before ovulation).
- **Day 14: ovulation**:
  - The LH surge causes the dominant follicle to release its egg.
  - The remaining follicle then becomes the corpus luteum.

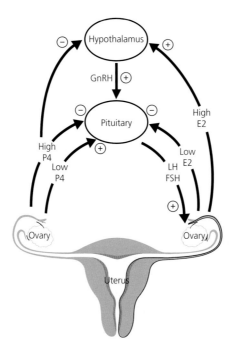

Fig. 11.1 Hypothalamic–pituitary–ovarian axis. GnRH, gonadotrophin-releasing hormone; FSH, follicle-stimulating hormone; LH, luteinizing hormone; E2, oestrogen; P4, progesterone.

- **Days 15–28: luteal/secretory phase**:
  - The corpus luteum starts to produce oestrogen and progesterone (but relatively more progesterone).
  - Increasing progesterone levels causes secretory changes to the endometrium.
  - Progesterone has an inhibitory effect on the secretion of FSH and LH.

MICRO-facts

Peak progesterone level is reached midway through the luteal phase (usually around day 21).

- If the egg is not fertilized, the corpus luteum begins to degenerate.
- This causes a fall in oestrogen and progesterone levels.
- Without the support of oestrogen and progesterone, the endometrium begins to break down and the whole cycle starts again (see Fig. 11.2).

Gynaecology

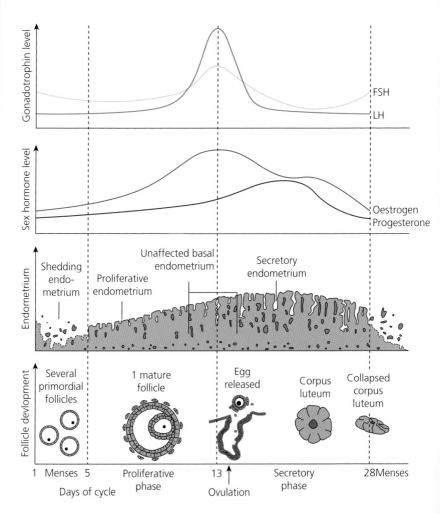

Fig. 11.2 **The menstrual cycle.**

11.2 AMENORRHOEA

- **Definitions:**
  - **Primary amenorrhoea:** menstruation has not started by the age of 16 years **or** failure to develop secondary sexual characteristics by the age of 14 years.
  - **Secondary amenorrhoea:** absence of periods for at least 6 months in a woman who had previously been menstruating.

Causes of amenorrhoea

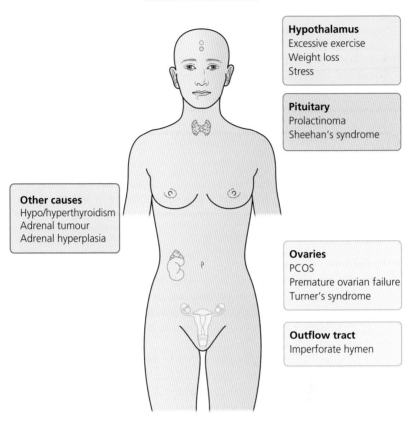

Fig. 11.3 Causes of amenorrhoea. PCOS, polycystic ovary syndrome.

MICRO-facts

Turner's syndrome

- 45 XO genotype.
- Causes primary amenorrhoea.
- Clinical features:
    - short stature;
    - webbed neck;
    - normal intelligence;
    - broad chest with widely spaced nipples.

continued...

Gynaecology

continued...

- The hypothalamus and pituitary function normally, but the streak ovaries are incapable of producing oestrogen, resulting in poor secondary sexual characteristics.
- Follicle-stimulating hormone and luteinizing hormone levels will be markedly elevated (owing to the lack of negative feedback from oestrogen).

MICRO-print
Sheehan's syndrome
This is hypopituitarism due to pituitary necrosis as a result of severe postpartum haemorrhage. It usually presents as failure to lactate.

POLYCYSTIC OVARY SYNDROME

- **Definition**:
  - A diagnosis of polycystic ovary syndrome (PCOS) is made when at least two of the following criteria are met:
    - Polycystic ovary on ultrasound: usually multiple (≥ 12) small follicles, each measuring 2–9 mm in diameter and/or ovarian volume > 10 mL.
    - Irregular periods: usually > 5 weeks apart.
    - Hyperandrogenism (clinically and/or biochemically):
      ○ clinically: hirsutism (acne/excess body hair);
      ○ biochemically: raised serum testosterone with low steroid hormone-binding globulin (SHBG).
- **Epidemiology**:
  - affects around 5–10% of women of reproductive age;
  - common cause of anovulatory infertility.

MICRO-facts
Polycystic ovary syndrome tends to be overdiagnosed and over/poorly treated.

- **Pathophysiology**:
  - The pathophysiology of PCOS remains unclear.
  - It is likely to be multifactorial:
    - Genetics.
    - Insulin resistance (with compensatory hyperinsulinaemia):

○ increases adrenal androgen production;
○ reduces hepatic production of SHBG.
- Raised LH level:
  ○ increases ovarian androgen production.
- Usually there is an increased serum free androgen level.
- The effect of this increased free androgen depends on where it is:
  - Intra-ovarian:
    ○ disrupts formation of follicles;
    ○ causes irregular or absent ovulation.
  - Peripherally:
    ○ hirsutism.
- **Clinical features**:
  - none in some cases;
  - subfertility;
  - amenorrhoea or oligomenorrhoea (infrequent periods);
  - hirsutism;
  - miscarriage;
  - obesity (can be a cause or effect of the disease).
- **Investigations**:
  - Blood tests:
    - testosterone: ↑;
    - SHBG: ↓;
    - LH: ↑;
    - FSH: normal;
    - prolactin: may be normal or slightly ↑ (also useful in excluding prolactinoma);
    - thyroid-stimulating hormone: to assess thyroid function.
  - Transvaginal ultrasound scan of ovaries:
    - to assess ovarian volume and presence of multiple, small follicles.

MICRO-facts

It is worth noting that women with polycystic ovary syndrome (PCOS) may not have all of these test results. Remember that PCOS can be diagnosed without blood tests.

- **Management**:
  - Hirsutism:
    - Co-cyprindiol (which contains an anti-androgen) (Dianette®).
    - Combined oral contraceptive pill containing an anti-androgen (Yasmin®).
    - Can get topical anti-androgens for acne (Vaniqa®).

- Subfertility:
    - Diet and exercise to reduce weight.
    - Metformin:
        ○ can help reduce insulin levels;
        ○ may restore ovulation;
        ○ however, there are no trials to prove its effectiveness.
    - Inducing ovulation (see later).
- **Complications**:
    - type 2 diabetes mellitus;
    - gestational diabetes.

11.3 INFERTILITY

- **Definition**:
    - failure to conceive after regular unprotected sexual intercourse for 2 years in the absence of known reproductive pathology;
    - **primary infertility**: for couples who have never conceived;
    - **secondary infertility**: for couples who have previously conceived.
- **Epidemiology**:
    - Ovarian failure and tubal damage (due to infection) are the most common causes of infertility in women.
    - The commonest cause of infertility in men is abnormal semen.

FEMALE INFERTILITY

- **Anovulation**:
    - Ovulation is detected by an elevated mid-luteal-phase serum progesterone level (usually at day 21 in a 28 day cycle).

> **MICRO-facts**
>
> The luteal phase is always fixed at 14 days from the end of a cycle. Therefore, the best method to calculate the mid-luteal phase is to subtract 7 days from the length of the cycle. For example:
> - mid-luteal phase for a 28 day cycle is day 21;
> - mid-luteal phase for a 35 day cycle is day 28.

- Causes:
    - hypothalamic hypogonadism;
    - hyperprolactinaemia;
    - PCOS;
    - hypo/hyperthyroidism;
    - premature ovarian failure.

- **Problems with fertilization**:
  - The following can cause fallopian tube damage and blockage:
    - pelvic inflammatory disease (see Chapter 19, Genital tract infections);
    - endometriosis (see Chapter 13, Benign gynaecological disease);
    - previous pelvic surgery (e.g. appendicitis) resulting in adhesion formation.

MICRO-facts

Patency of the fallopian tubes can be assessed by the following methods:

- Hysterosalpingogram (HSG):
  - radio-opaque contrast is injected through the cervix;
  - spillage from the tubes, indicating patency, can be visualized on a radiograph.
- Laparoscopy and dye test:
  - dye is injected through the cervix and spillage is identified during laparoscopy.
- Transvaginal ultrasound with ultrasound-opaque liquid:
  - similar to HSG.

- **Problems with implantation**:
  - Causes:
    - fibroids.

MALE INFERTILITY

- **Semen analysis**:
  - Sample should be provided by masturbation after 2–7 days of sexual abstinence.
  - Normal values:
    - volume: >2 mL;
    - sperm count: >20 million/mL;
    - motility: $>50\%$.
  - Abnormal semen analysis:
    - oligospermia: <20 million/mL;
    - severe oligospermia: <5 million/mL;
    - azoospermia: no sperm detected.
- **Causes of abnormal semen analysis**:
  - Idiopathic.
  - Drug exposure:
    - alcohol;
    - smoking (especially cannabis);

- anabolic steroids;
- solvents.
- Anti-sperm antibodies:
  - causes clumping of sperm and poor motility.
- Infections:
  - epididymitis;
  - mumps orchitis.

INDUCING OVULATION

- **Lifestyle advice**:
  - weight restoration may restore ovulation in hypothalamic hypogonadism.
- **Clomifene**:
  - first-line drug for inducing ovulation in PCOS;
  - used for about 6 months;
  - it is an anti-oestrogen and therefore promotes the release of FSH and LH;
  - ultrasound monitoring should be used to reduce the risk of multiple pregnancy;
  - metformin increases the effectiveness of clomifene.
- **Gonadotrophin therapy**:
  - used for PCOS if clomifene fails or in hypothalamic hypogonadism with normal weight;
  - recombinant FSH is given subcutaneously each day;
  - ultrasound is used to monitor follicle development;
  - once a follicle is mature and an appropriate size, recombinant LH is given.
- **Ovarian diathermy**:
  - laparoscopic procedure;
  - each ovary is diathermied in a few locations.
- **Bromocriptine**:
  - used for hyperprolactinaemia;
  - as a dopamine agonist, it has an inhibitory effect on the release of prolactin.

ASSISTED CONCEPTION

- **Intra-uterine insemination**:
  - placement of the sperm sample into the uterus during ovulation;
  - ovulation is usually stimulated with gonadotrophins;
  - can only be considered if the fallopian tubes are patent;
  - live birth rate is around 10% per cycle.

- **Tubal surgery**:
  - patency and tubal function can be restored to allow natural conception.
- ***In vitro* fertilization** (IVF):
  - In women <36 years old, the live birth rate can be 35% per cycle.
  - IVF is not as effective over the age of 38:
    - oocyte donation is suggested at such ages.

MICRO-print

A typical ***in vitro* fertilization (IVF) cycle** will include the following:

- Pituitary downregulation with gonadotrophin-releasing hormone agonists, which will prevent the normal luteinizing hormone surge (and ovulation) during ovarian stimulation.
- Ovarian stimulation with gonadotrophins.
- Ovulation triggered by human chorionic gonadotrophin.
- Oocyte collection.
- Insemination of oocytes (sperm is mixed with oocytes and incubated).
- Embryos are chosen and transferred to the uterus. If <40 years old, a maximum of two embryos can be transferred. If >40 years old, up to three embryos can be used.
- Luteal support with progesterone.
- See also: http://www.nhs.uk/Conditions/IVF/Pages/How-is-it-performed.aspx

---

- **Intra-cytoplasmic sperm injection**:
  - this method involves injecting a single sperm into the cytoplasm of the oocyte;
  - can be used during IVF;
  - useful when sperm have poor motility.
- **Oocyte ('egg') donation**:
  - Donors undergo an IVF cycle and their oocytes are retrieved.
  - These oocytes are then fertilized with sperm from the recipient woman's partner.
  - The endometrium of the recipient woman is prepared with oestrogen and progesterone.
  - The embryos are then transferred to the recipient woman.
- **Surrogacy**:
  - Straight surrogacy:
    - the surrogate's oocytes are fertilized with the commissioning woman's partner's sperm.

Gynaecology

- Host surrogacy:
  - the commissioning woman undergoes IVF so that her oocytes can be collected;
  - these are fertilized with her partner's sperm and then transferred to the surrogate's uterus.

MICRO-reference

National Institute for Health and Clinical Excellence. Fertility: assessment and treatment of people with fertility problems. NICE Clinical Guideline 11. London, UK: NICE, 2004. Available at: http://www.rcog.org.uk/files/rcog-corp/uploaded-files/NEBFertilitySummary.pdf

---

11.4 MENOPAUSE

- **Definitions**:
  - Menopause:
    - Permanent cessation of menstruation owing to the loss of ovarian function.
    - There needs to be 12 consecutive months of amenorrhoea before this term can be used.
    - The average age when this happens is 52 years.
  - Peri-menopause:
    - This describes the time leading up to the menopause. It starts when features of the approaching menopause (e.g. menstrual irregularity) are first noticed and ends 12 months after the last period.
  - Premature menopause:
    - Menopause occurring before the age of 40 years.
    - Causes:
      - surgical (removal of ovaries);
      - autoimmune;
      - chemotherapy/radiotherapy to pelvis;
      - infections.
- **Clinical features**:
  - These are related to oestrogen deficiency.

MICRO-print

Oestrogen has an influence on the rate of bone turnover. It normally maintains the balance between bone resorption and bone formation.

This balance is disturbed when there is loss of circulating oestrogen (menopause). The rate of bone turnover increases, with faster bone resorption than bone formation.

All of this compromises bone strength and increases the risk of fractures.

Gynaecology

- Vasomotor problems:
  - hot flushes;
  - night sweats.
- Vaginal atrophy:
  - dyspareunia (pain during intercourse);
  - itching;
  - burning;
  - dryness.
- Urinary symptoms:
  - frequency;
  - urgency;
  - nocturia;
  - incontinence.
- Psychological symptoms:
  - mood swings;
  - anxiety;
  - forgetfulness;
  - poor concentration.
- Late effects of oestrogen deficiency:
  - osteoporosis and bony fractures;
  - cardiac disease;
  - cerebrovascular disease.
- **Investigations**:
  - Diagnosis is made clinically:
    - FSH is usually high, released in boluses and causes peripheral vasodilatation, leading to the hot sweats;
    - thyroid function tests: thyroid disease may present similarly and should be excluded.
- **Management**:
  - Hormone replacement therapy (HRT):
    - Oestrogen-only regimen:
      ○ can be given to women who have had a hysterectomy;
      ○ avoid in women with a previous history of endometriosis.
    - Oestrogen and progesterone regimen (combined HRT):
      ○ this regimen is used for women who still have a uterus;
      ○ can be cyclical or continuous;
      ○ unopposed oestrogen may lead to endometrial hyperplasia/carcinoma;
      ○ adding progesterone helps to reduce this risk.

Gynaecology

> **MICRO-print**
> - Cyclical combined hormone replacement therapy:
>   - Progesterone is only given at fixed intervals, e.g. for 10–14 days every 4 weeks.
>   - This will result in cyclical bleeding.
> - Continuous combined HRT:
>   - Progesterone is given continuously, leading to amenorrhoea.
>   - This is not suitable for use until the woman has been period free for 12 months.

- Topical oestrogen regimen:
  - can be used for women who have only urogenital symptoms.
- Duration of treatment:
  - Treating menopausal symptoms:
    - HRT can be used for up to 5 years and then stopped for review.
  - Treating/preventing osteoporosis:
    - may wish to switch to other agents such as bisphosphonates;
    - may benefit from bone densiometry to assess the degree of osteoporosis and then plan management depending on the result.
  - Premature menopause:
    - HRT until the average age of menopause (around 52 years).

Table 11.1 Benefits and risks of hormone replacement therapy (HRT).

BENEFITS OF HRT	RISKS OF HRT
Relief from hot flushes	Increased risk of gallbladder disease
Relief from vaginal dryness	Increased risk of venous thromboembolism
Improvement in urinary symptoms	Slight increased risk of breast cancer (if on combined HRT)
Reduces risk of osteoporotic fractures	Increased risk of endometrial cancer (if oestrogen is unopposed)

Table 11.2 Modes of delivering hormone replacement therapy.

OESTROGEN	PROGESTERONE
Oral	Oral
Transdermal (patch)	Transdermal (patch)
Subcutaneous (implant)	Directly into uterus (intra-uterine system)
Topical	

Disorders of the menstrual cycle

12.1 HEAVY MENSTRUAL BLEEDING

- **Definitions**:
  - Heavy menstrual bleeding (HMB; menorrhagia) should be defined **subjectively** as excessive menstrual blood loss that interferes with a woman's physical, emotional, social or material quality of life.
  - Dysfunctional uterine bleeding (DUB) is abnormal bleeding from the genital tract in the absence of any demonstrable pathology.
- **Epidemiology**:
  - 5% of women aged 30–49 consult their GPs every year with HMB.
  - It is the indication for over half of the hysterectomies performed.
- **Aetiology**:
  - **Idiopathic**: in the majority of cases there is no identifiable cause for HMB; this is called DUB.
  - **Pelvic pathology**:
    - The most common identified causes of HMB are:
      ○ **uterine fibroids**;
      ○ **uterine polyps**.
    - These increase the endometrial surface.

MICRO-print

Objectively, heavy menstrual bleeding (HMB) is defined as menstrual blood loss >80 mL per period. This is the maximum volume of blood that can be lost in one period without causing iron-deficiency anaemia. However, measuring menstrual blood loss is impractical. HMB should be assessed subjectively.

    - Less commonly, it may be a presentation of:
      ○ chronic pelvic inflammatory disease (PID);
      ○ endometriosis;
      ○ adenomyosis;
      ○ endometrial hyperplasia or carcinoma;
      ○ cervical malignancy.

- **Iatrogenic** factors may be implicated:
  - Intra-uterine contraceptive device (IUCD).
  - Anti-coagulation therapy.
- Rarely, the cause is **systemic**:
  - Coagulopathies, e.g. von Willebrand's disease.
  - Hypothyroidism.
- **Clinical features**:
  - **History**:
    - Establish **amount of bleeding**:
      - do you use tampons or towels, or both?
      - how often do you have to change tampons/towels?
      - have you experienced passing **clots** or **flooding**? These are indicative of heavy blood loss;
      - impact on lifestyle;
      - time course of symptoms.
    - **Related symptoms** may indicate underlying pelvic pathology:
      - irregular bleeding;
      - inter-menstrual bleeding (IMB);
      - post-coital bleeding;
      - pelvic pain;
      - timing of pain, and whether it is cyclical;
      - dyspareunia; may be associated with endometriosis or chronic PID.
    - Vaginal discharge.
    - Symptoms of anaemia.
- **Examination**:
  - Often unremarkable.
  - Mass:
    - fibroids may present as an irregular pelvic mass;
    - ovarian mass.
  - Tenderness:
    - endometriosis;
    - adenomyosis ($\pm$ enlarged uterus).
  - A fixed, retroverted uterus or adnexae:
    - may indicate endometriosis.
- **Investigations**:
  - All women should have a **full blood count** to exclude iron-deficiency anaemia.
  - If the history and examination are suggestive of a systemic disorder, conduct the relevant investigations, e.g. thyroid function tests.
  - If a structural abnormality is suspected, further investigation is needed (see Fig. 12.1).
  - Endometrial biopsy should be considered.

Gynaecology

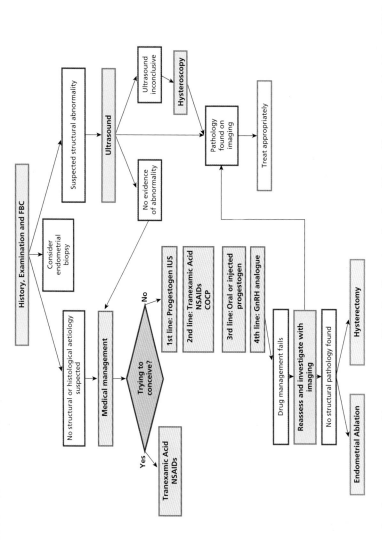

Fig. 12.1 Algorithm for the management of heavy menstrual bleeding (based on data from National Institute for Health and Clinical Excellence, Clinical Guidance 44). Note that, in practice, the second-line treatments are often trialled before the intra-uterine system. COCP, combined oral contraceptive pill; FBC, full blood count; GnRH, gonadotrophin-releasing hormone; NSAID, non-steroidal anti-inflammatory drug.

Table 12.1 Medical management of heavy menstrual bleeding (adapted from data from National Institute for Health and Clinical Excellence, Clinical Guidance 44).

	TREATMENT	MECHANISM	CONTRACEPTIVE?	ADVANTAGES	DISADVANTAGES
First-line	Progestogen intra-uterine system	Prevents endometrial proliferation	Yes	No effect on future fertility	May cause irregular bleeding for up to 6 months (for side-effects, see Table 18.4)
Second-line	Tranexamic acid	Oral anti-fibrinolytic	No	No effect on future fertility	May cause indigestion, diarrhoea or headache
	Oral NSAIDs, e.g. mefenamic acid	Reduces prostaglandin production	No	No effect on future fertility Relieves dysmenorrhoea	May cause indigestion, diarrhoea Contraindicated in asthma, peptic ulcer disease
	COCP	Prevents endometrial proliferation	Yes	No effect on future fertility	See Table 18.1

(Continued)

Table 12.1 (*Continued*)

	TREATMENT	MECHANISM	CONTRACEPTIVE?	ADVANTAGES	DISADVANTAGES
Third-line	Oral or injected progestogen	Prevents endometrial proliferation	Yes, although oral progestogen is not licensed as such	No effect on future fertility	Oral: weight gain, bloating, breast tenderness and acne Injected: see Tables 18.2 and 18.3
Other	GnRH analogue	Prevents oestrogen and progesterone release	No. Although they inhibit ovulation, they are not licensed as contraceptives because of side-effects, e.g. bone loss	No effect on future fertility	Menopausal-like symptoms HRT is recommended if used for >6 months

COCP, combined oral contraceptive pill; GnRH, gonadotrophin-releasing hormone; HRT, hormone replacement therapy; NSAID, non-steroidal anti-inflammatory drug.

Table 12.2 Surgical management of heavy menstrual bleeding (HMB) (adapted on data from National Institute for Health and Clinical Excellence, Clinical Guidance 44).

	INDICATION	MECHANISM	ADVANTAGES	COMPLICATIONS
Endometrial ablation	Consider before hysterectomy in women with only HMB and a uterine size ≤10 week pregnancy	Destruction of the basal endometrium prevents regeneration and menstruation	Fewer complications than hysterectomy	Impact on fertility: pregnancy is unlikely but contraception is still required Vaginal discharge, increased menstrual pain and cramping are common Further surgery may be required if unsuccessful
Hysterectomy	Consider when other HMB treatments have failed, are contraindicated or refused	Surgical removal of the uterus	Amenorrhoea	Infection Haemorrhage Damage to bladder/bowel Urinary dysfunction May affect sexual function

MICRO-facts

Indications for endometrial biopsy (National Institute for Health and Clinical Excellence, Clinical Guidance 44)

- Heavy menstrual bleeding (HMB) with persistent inter-menstrual bleeding.
- Increased endometrial thickness on ultrasound.
- HMB in women > 45 years (in practice, many gynaecologists use 35 years).
- Pharmaceutical treatment has failed or been ineffective.

- **Management**:
  - See Fig. 12.1; Tables 12.1 and 12.2.
  - National Institute for Health and Clinical Excellence guidelines recommend that two medical treatments should be used before considering surgery.

MICRO-reference

National Institute for Health and Clinical Excellence. Heavy menstrual bleeding. NICE Clinical Guidance 44. London, UK: NICE, 2007. Available at http://guidance.nice.org.uk/CG44/Guidance/pdf/English

MICRO-print
When should the ovaries be removed too?

For women over 55 years undergoing total abdominal hysterectomy (TAH), bilateral salpingo-oophorectomy (BSO) is routine. In younger women the evidence is less clear. The decision should be made on an individual basis.

- Benefits of simultaneous BSO include:
  - prevents ovarian cancer;
  - prevents symptoms related to retained ovaries, e.g. pain;
  - oophorectomy post-TAH is a difficult operation; BSO is more straightforward when carried out with TAH.
- Disadvantages:
  - BSO induces an early menopause, so the beneficial effects of oestrogen on bone and the cardiovascular system are lost; although oestrogen may be replaced with hormone replacement therapy, this carries its own risks;
- The following are also considered:
  - the patient's family history of ovarian and breast cancer;
  - any intrinsic problems with the ovary at the time of the procedure.

Gynaecology

MICRO-case

A 40-year-old woman was referred to the gynaecology department by her GP with a 2 year history of heavy menstrual bleeding (HMB). Her periods were irregular; she was bleeding for 10 days in a 20 day cycle. When bleeding, she needed to change tampons hourly and wore a pad for extra protection. She had also experienced several episodes of flooding, which were particularly distressing. She denied inter-menstrual and post-coital bleeding, dyspareunia and vaginal discharge.

The patient had two children aged 10 and 7. She had no other significant past medical, gynaecological or obstetric history.

Bimanual and speculum examination were unremarkable. A full blood count revealed a microcytic anaemia; she was taking ferrous sulphate.

To date, her GP had tried several medical treatments. There was no improvement with the intra-uterine system, which was removed. She had been taking the combined oral contraceptive pill, tranexamic acid and mefenamic acid for over 6 months. These had not reduced her bleeding.

Given the failure of medical treatment, the gynaecologist ordered a pelvic ultrasound, which was unremarkable, and an endometrial biopsy, which was negative. The gynaecologist discussed the options for surgical management with the patient, who later underwent endometrial ablation. Post-surgery, her HMB improved but she experienced painful menstrual cramps. She will be followed up to monitor her symptoms; ultimately she may need a hysterectomy.

Key points:

- In many cases, no underlying pathology is found for HMB. This is called dysfunctional uterine bleeding.
- HMB can have a significant impact on a woman's quality of life.
- Failure of drug treatment is an indication for endometrial biopsy.
- Increased menstrual pain is a common complication of endometrial ablation.

12.2 DYSMENORRHOEA

- **Definition**:
  - Painful menstruation:
    - typically, a cramping lower abdominal pain that is associated with the onset of menstruation.
- **Epidemiology**:
  - very common; affects 50–90% of menstruating women;
  - 5–14% of women are frequently absent from work owing to dysmenorrhoea.

Table 12.3 A comparison of primary and secondary dysmenorrhoea.

	PRIMARY DYSMENORRHOEA	SECONDARY DYSMENORRHOEA
Onset	Typically, 6–12 months after menarche	Usually preceded by several years of painless periods
Timing and duration of pain	Shortly before menstruation begins, lasts up to 72 hours. Improves as menses ends	Not confined to menstruation. May be present throughout the menstrual cycle and exacerbated or relieved by menstruation
Associated symptoms	Non-gynaecological: • Nausea • Vomiting • Bloating • Migraine • Emotional symptoms	Gynaecological: • Dyspareunia • Inter-menstrual bleeding • Heavy menstrual bleeding • Vaginal discharge
Pelvic examination (perform in all women)	Normal	May be abnormal, e.g. pelvic/abdominal mass or tenderness
Investigations	Not required	May include ultrasound, endometrial biopsy or triple swabs
Treatment	NSAIDs and/or hormonal treatment, e.g. COCP	NSAIDs for pain relief + treatment of underlying cause

COCP, combined oral contraceptive pill; NSAID, non-steroidal anti-inflammatory drug.

- **Aetiology**:
  - Dysmenorrhoea may be:
    - **Primary**: there is no identifiable pelvic pathology.
    - **Secondary**: there is organic pelvic pathology:
      ○ endometriosis;
      ○ adenomyosis;
      ○ PID;
      ○ IUCD;
      ○ endometrial polyps;
      ○ fibroids.

12.3 POST-COITAL BLEEDING

- **Definition**:
  - non-menstrual vaginal bleeding immediately after sexual intercourse.
- **Aetiology**:
  - Cervical carcinoma.
  - Physiological: following first intercourse only.
  - From the vagina:
    - vaginitis, including atrophic vaginitis in post-menopausal women;
    - carcinoma.

> **MICRO-facts**
>
> **Cervical carcinoma** must be excluded in all women with **post-coital bleeding**.

  - From the cervix:
    - cervicitis;
    - trauma;
    - ectropion;
    - polyps.
- **Examination**:
  - bimanual;
  - speculum.
- **Investigations**:
  - cervical cytology with/without colposcopy;
  - triple swabs if indicated.
- **Management**:
  - treatment of underlying pathology.

12.4 IRREGULAR AND INTER-MENSTRUAL BLEEDING

- **Definitions**:
  - Normal menstruation:
    - cycle length 23–35 days;
    - menstruation <8 days;
    - no IMB.
  - 'Irregular' periods may be too frequent, infrequent or of variable length:
    - cycle length is shorter or longer than 23–35 days;
    - cycle length varies by >7 days between the shortest and longest cycle.

- Oligomenorrhoea:
  - infrequent periods: a cycle may last between 35 days and 6 months.
- Inter-menstrual bleeding:
  - bleeding between periods.

MICRO-facts

Women may not be able to distinguish between irregular periods and inter-menstrual bleeding.

- **Aetiology**:
  - Anovulation:
    - Frequent and/or prolonged periods are likely to be caused by anovulatory cycles. This is common around menarche and menopause.
  - Pelvic pathology:
    - Ectropion.
    - Fibroid uterus:
      ○ note that fibroids increase the endometrial area. Bleeding is not from the fibroids per se.
    - Uterine/cervical polyps.
    - Adenomyosis.
    - Ovarian cysts.
    - PID.
    - **Malignancy**:
      ○ endometrial;
      ○ cervical.
  - Contraception:
    - Combined oral contraceptive pill (COCP):
      ○ breakthrough bleeding is caused by under-dosing, or by interaction with drugs that induce hepatic enzyme activity, e.g. carbamazepine.
    - IUCD.
    - Progesterone-only pill.
    - Progesterone injection.
  - Thyroid disease.
- **Clinical features**:
  - History:
    - age;
    - related menstrual symptoms;
    - contraception;
    - onset and duration of IMB: suspect malignancy with recent IMB in older women.

Gynaecology

- Examination:
  - body mass index;
  - speculum;
  - bimanual.
- **Investigations**:
  - As for HMB.
  - Exclude malignancy in the older woman:
    - Endometrial biopsy:
      - ○ persistent IMB with HMB is an indication for biopsy.
    - Cervical cytology.
- **Management**:
  - treat underlying pathology;
  - irregular bleeding and IMB without underlying pathology are considered the result of anovulatory cycles; they may be treated with the intra-uterine system or COCP.

12.5 PRE-MENSTRUAL SYNDROME

- **Definition**:
  - The regular occurrence of cyclical psychological, physical and behavioural symptoms during the luteal phase of the menstrual cycle that are significantly improved or resolved by the end of menstruation.
- **Epidemiology**:
  - Mild pre-menstrual syndrome (PMS) is very common: 13% of working women take time off each year due to PMS;
  - In 5% of women, symptoms are severe.
- **Clinical features**:
  - Psychological:
    - mood swings;
    - depressed mood;
    - irritability;
    - anxiety;
    - decreased libido.
  - Physical:
    - bloating;
    - mastalgia;
    - abdominal cramps;
    - headache;
    - cyclical weight gain.
  - Behavioural:
    - poor concentration;
    - aggression.

MICRO-facts

Pre-menstrual syndrome may be mild, moderate or severe:

- **Mild**: symptoms do not interfere with lifestyle.
- **Moderate**: symptoms interfere with lifestyle.
- **Severe**: loss of normal function; withdrawal from social and professional activities.

- **Aetiology**:
  - Unclear. Cyclical ovarian activity and serotonin levels may be implicated.
- **Management**:
  - confirm diagnosis with a symptom diary;
  - selective serotonin re-uptake inhibitors, e.g. fluoxetine;
  - COCP;
  - cognitive–behavioural therapy may improve anxiety, mood and behavioural problems;
  - non-steroidal anti-inflammatory drugs for physical symptoms;
  - complementary therapies, e.g. relaxation.

MICRO-reference

Royal College of Obstetricians and Gynaecologists. Management of premenstrual syndrome. London, UK: RCOG, 2007. Available at http://www.rcog.org.uk/files/rcog-corp/uploaded-files/GT48ManagementPremensturalSyndrome.pdf

Gynaecology

13 Benign gynaecological disease

13.1 ENDOMETRIOSIS

- **Definition**:
  - Deposits of endometrial-like tissue outside the uterine cavity, which cause chronic inflammation.
  - The most common sites of endometrial deposits are within the pelvis:
    - peritoneum;
    - uterosacral ligaments;
    - pouch of Douglas;
    - rectovaginal septum (fascia between the vagina and rectum);
    - ovaries.

> **MICRO-print**
>
> Rarely, endometrial deposits may be found outside of the pelvis. Deposits in the pleura may present with cyclical haemoptysis or haemopneumothorax.

> **MICRO-facts**
>
> **Endometriomas** or 'chocolate cysts' are ovarian cysts lined internally with ectopic endometrium. Menstrual bleeds lead to the accumulation of dark brown fluid within the cyst. The destruction of ovarian tissue that accompanies endometrioma formation may also contribute to subfertility.

- **Epidemiology**:
  - it is estimated that 2–22% of women may have endometriosis.
- **Aetiology**:
  - The precise aetiology is unknown, although it is likely to be multifactorial.
  - There are several hypotheses:
    - retrograde menstruation: the flow of menstrual fluid back through the fallopian tubes allows endometrial tissue to implant ectopically;
    - metaplasia of peritoneal cells into endometrial tissue;

- haematogenous or lymphatic spread;
- implantation into surgical scars.
- However, none of these hypotheses can singularly explain the development of endometriosis in all known sites.
- **Pathophysiology**:
  - like normal endometrium, ectopic endometrial deposits are oestrogen dependent;
  - cyclical withdrawal bleeds cause local inflammation and pain;
  - inflammation may result in pelvic adhesions and fibrosis, leading to anatomical distortion and subfertility.

MICRO-facts
Symptoms decrease during pregnancy and after the menopause because deposits of endometriosis are oestrogen dependent.

- **Clinical features**:
  - **History**:
    - Pain:
      - chronic pelvic pain;
      - secondary dysmenorrhoea;
      - deep dyspareunia;
      - ovulatory pain;
      - painful caesarean section scar.
    - Cyclical or perimenstrual bladder and bowel symptoms:
      - pain/difficulty in passing stools;
      - painful micturition;
      - rectal bleeding;
      - haematuria.
    - Subfertility.
    - Chronic fatigue.
    - Deposits of endometriosis may be asymptomatic, found incidentally, e.g. during laparoscopic sterilization.
  - **Examination**:
    - Often normal in mild and moderate disease.
    - **Bimanual**:
      - localized pelvic tenderness;
      - thickening behind the uterus or in the adnexae;
      - fixed and retroverted uterus;
      - tender uterosacral ligaments;
      - enlarged ovaries;
      - palpable, tender nodules.

Gynaecology

- **Speculum**:
  - ○ visible nodules on the vagina or cervix.
- **Investigations**.
  - Direct visualization of the pelvis by laparoscopy is the gold standard for diagnosis. Suspicious lesions are biopsied.

MICRO-print

Laparoscopically, deposits of endometriosis may appear as:

- red haemorrhagic spots;
- white scars/brown spots ('powder burn');
- adhesions.

Endometriomas may also be seen.

  - Transvaginal ultrasound scan (TVS) may be used to diagnose endometriomas.
  - Serum CA-125 is a biomarker that may be raised in malignancy (including ovarian and uterine cancer) and in benign conditions. Although CA-125 may be significantly raised in endometriosis, it is not a useful diagnostic test.
- **Differential diagnosis**:
  - adenomyosis;
  - fibroids;
  - primary dysmenorrhoea;
  - interstitial cystitis;
  - chronic pelvic inflammatory disease;
  - irritable bowel syndrome (IBS);
  - pelvic masses, e.g. malignancies.
- **Management**:
  - **Medical**:
    - **First-line**: non-steroidal anti-inflammatory drug.
    - **Second-line**: paracetamol.
    - **Third-line**: codeine.
    - **Hormonal treatment**: for pain relief if analgesics are insufficient.
      - ○ **combined oral contraceptive pill**: up to six pill packets can be taken back-to-back to reduce the pain on withdrawal bleeding;
      - ○ **progestogens** may be taken continually or cyclically;
      - ○ **gonadotrophin-releasing hormone (GnRH) analogues** ($\pm$ 'add-back' oestrogen and progestogen to protect against loss of bone mineral density);
      - ○ the complications and side-effect profiles of these drugs are described in Chapter 18, Contraception.

MICRO-facts

Hormonal treatments do not improve fertility. Symptoms often recur once the treatment is stopped.

- **Surgical**:
  - **Laparoscopic laser ablation** of endometriotic deposits reduces pain and improves fertility.
  - **Adhesiolysis** (dissection of adhesions) reduces pain and improves fertility.
  - If other treatment fails, **total abdominal hysterectomy** (TAH) with/without bilateral salpingo-oophorectomy (BSO) may be carried out in women who have completed their family. Combined hormone replacement therapy (HRT) is given if BSO is carried out.
  - Because of the adhesions present, surgery may be difficult. There is a risk of damage to surrounding structures.
- **Endometriomas**:
  - Suspected endometriomas (identified on TVS) are managed as a suspected ovarian malignancy (see later under Benign conditions of the ovaries).
  - Laparoscopic ovarian cystectomy of confirmed endometriomas reduces recurrence and pain, and improves fertility.
- **Treatment of subfertility**:
  - Medical treatment does not improve fertility outcomes.
  - Surgical ablation and adhesiolysis improve fertility outcomes.
  - Tubal flushing is also effective.
  - In more severe disease, intra-uterine insemination and *in vitro* fertilization are used.
- **Prognosis**:
  - Relapse is common following medical and surgical treatment. Up to 50% of women require further intervention.
  - The success of fertility treatment is multifactorial, depending largely on the severity of disease.

MICRO-reference

Royal College of Obstetricians and Gynaecologists. The investigation and management of endometriosis. Green Top Guideline no. 24. London, UK: RCOG, 2006. Available at http://www.rcog.org.uk/files/rcog-corp/uploaded-files/GT24InvestigationEndometriosis2006.pdf

Gynaecology

MICRO-case

A 35-year-old nulliparous woman was referred to gynaecology by her GP with a 12 month history of intermittent pelvic pain and deep dyspareunia. She also described a 5 year history of dysmenorrhoea. She denied any bladder or bowel symptoms. She and her husband are trying for a baby.

On bimanual examination the uterus was fixed and retroverted. There was thickening and tenderness in the adnexae. Speculum examination was unremarkable.

The GP had ordered a transvaginal scan, which was unremarkable. A 12 month course of ibuprofen and paracetamol had not relieved her symptoms. Hormonal treatment was unacceptable because of her wish to conceive.

Diagnostic laparoscopy was conducted. Endometriotic deposits were visualized on the uterosacral ligaments and peritoneum. These were biopsied and ablated. Post-laparoscopy the patient described moderate relief of her pain. She will be followed-up to monitor potential subfertility and symptom recurrence.

Key points:

- Endometriosis is most commonly diagnosed in women aged 30–40 years.
- Often, examination in endometriosis is normal. The examination findings in this case are suggestive of endometriosis but not pathognomonic.
- As relapse is common, patients may require further intervention.

13.2 ADENOMYOSIS

- **Definition**:
  - the presence of endometrial glands and stroma within the myometrium.
- **Epidemiology**:
  - the incidence is unknown;
  - usually presents in multiparous women in their late thirties and early forties.
- **Aetiology**:
  - unknown;
  - uterine damage during pregnancy, parturition or surgery may be a risk factor.
- **Clinical features**:
  - **History**:
    - heavy menstrual bleeding;
    - secondary dysmenorrhoea;

- dyspareunia;
- subfertility;
- also commonly asymptomatic.
- **Examination**:
  - symmetrically enlarged, 'bulky' uterus;
  - uterus may be tender.
- **Investigations**:
  - MRI and TVS may help to diagnose adenomyosis pre-operatively;
  - however, a definitive diagnosis is made histologically, post-hysterectomy.
- **Differential diagnosis**:
  - fibroids;
  - endometriosis;
  - chronic pelvic pain.
- **Management**:
  - **Medical**:
    - as for the treatment of heavy menstrual bleeding (see Table 12.1). GnRH analogues may be effective in relieving pain.
  - **Surgical**:
    - TAH with/without BSO.

13.3 CHRONIC PELVIC PAIN

- **Definition**:
  - Intermittent or constant pain in the lower abdomen or pelvis **lasting at least 6 months** which **does not occur exclusively with menstruation or intercourse,** and is not associated with pregnancy.

> **MICRO-reference**
> Royal College of Obstetricians and Gynaecologists. The initial management of chronic pelvic pain. Green Top Guideline no. 41. London, UK: RCOG, 2005. Available at http://www.rcog.org.uk/womens-health/clinical-guidance/initial-management-chronic-pelvic-pain-green-top-41

- **Epidemiology**:
  - affects 16% of women.
- **Aetiology**:
  - endometriosis;
  - adenomyosis;
  - pelvic adhesions;

- IBS;
- interstitial cystitis;
- psychological.

MICRO-facts

In many women, an underlying pathology is not found.

- **Investigations**:
  - TVS;
  - MRI;
  - laparoscopy.
- **Management**:
  - treatment of the underlying cause;
  - analgesia and chronic pain management.

13.4 FIBROIDS

- **Definition**:
  - fibroids, also known as leiomyomata, are benign tumours of the myometrium.
- **Epidemiology**:
  - One of the most common gynaecological problems affecting women in the UK.
  - More common in:
    - women approaching the menopause;
    - Afro-Caribbean women;
    - women with a family history of fibroids.

MICRO-reference

National Institute for Health and Clinical Excellence. Uterine embolisation for fibroids. London, UK: NICE, 2010. Available at http://www.nice.org.uk/nicemedia/live/11025/51706/51706.pdf

---

- **Pathophysiology**:
  - Fibroids are formed from smooth muscle and fibrous elements.
  - They vary in size from a few millimetres in diameter to tumours that fill the whole abdomen.
  - Fibroids may be classified by their site into: intra-mural, subserosal, submucosal and cervical. Fibroids may also be pedunculated (see Fig.13.1).
  - Their growth is stimulated by oestrogen and progesterone.

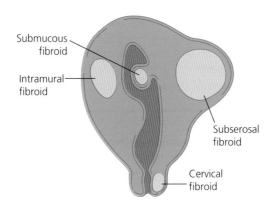

Fig. 13.1 The location of uterine fibroids.

- **Clinical features**:
  - History:
    - Asymptomatic:
      - in approximately 50% of cases;
      - often found incidentally.
    - Menorrhagia:
      - occurs in 30% of women;
      - more common with submucosal or intra-mural fibroids.
    - Dysmenorrhoea:
      - pain is rare unless torsion or red degeneration occur (see Complications).
    - Pressure effects:
      - frequency or urinary retention, if a large fibroid presses on the bladder;
      - hydronephrosis may occur, depending on the location of the fibroid, due to pressure on the ureter.
    - Infertility:
      - submucosal fibroids can cause distortion of the uterine cavity resulting in failure of implantation.
  - Examination:
    - Pelvic mass may be palpable on pelvic or abdominal palpation.
    - The mass is continuous with the uterus.
    - Single fibroids feel smooth.
    - Multiple fibroids feel irregular.
- **Investigations**:
  - Ultrasound scan.
  - Hysteroscopy:

- the uterus is insufflated with carbon dioxide or saline to allow visualization of the cavity, in order to assess for uterine distortion;
- general anaesthesia is not always required for this procedure.
- Full blood count:
  - heavy menstrual bleeding may cause anaemia.

MICRO-print

In some instances fibroids secrete erythropoietin, which causes poly-cythaemia. This is known as fibromatous erythrocytosis syndrome.

- **Treatment**:
  - Conservative:
    - If the fibroids are small or slow growing and the woman is asymptomatic, then no treatment is necessary.
    - Women with larger fibroids that are not removed may benefit from serial ultrasound in order to monitor growth.

MICRO-facts

Non-steroidal anti-inflammatory drugs and tranexamic acid are usually ineffective when menorrhagia occurs secondary to fibroids.

  - Medical:
    - GnRH agonists:
      ○ shrink the fibroid by inhibiting oestrogen and progesterone production;
      ○ cause menopausal side-effects;
      ○ increase the risk of osteoporosis; therefore, their use is limited to 6–9 months. The fibroids may grow back on stopping the treatment.
  - Surgical:
    - See Table 13.1.

MICRO-reference

Clinical Knowledge Summaries. Surgical treatment of fibroids. Available at http://www.cks.nhs.uk/fibroids#-411518

Table 13.1 Surgical treatment options for fibroids.

PROCEDURE	WHAT IT IS	FERTILITY CONSERVED?	COMPLICATIONS
Hysteroscopic removal of the fibroid	Usually performed on initial assessment of the uterine cavity. Submucosal fibroids may be resected	Yes	Uterine perforation and fluid overload (rare)
Myomectomy	Surgical removal of fibroids from the uterus. An abdominal approach, either open or laparoscopic is required to remove intra-mural and subserosal fibroids	Yes	Heavy blood loss (GnRH agonists are often used for 3 months prior in order to reduce the vascularity of the fibroid). Small fibroids may be missed
Uterine artery embolization	Injecting an embolic agent into the uterine arteries cuts off blood supply to the fibroid. Carried out by interventional radiologists	Not recommended in women who wish to conserve their fertility as a hysterectomy may still be required	Pain – a hysterectomy may be required to resolve the pain

(Continued)

Table 13.1 (*Continued*)

PROCEDURE	WHAT IT IS	FERTILITY CONSERVED?	COMPLICATIONS
Hysterectomy	Removal of the uterus with/without the ovaries and cervix, through either the vagina or abdomen (laparoscopic or open surgery)	No!	Mortality 1:1000 Haemorrhage Venous thromboembolic disease Pain Wound and chest infection GnRH, gonadotrophin-releasing hormone.

- **Complications**:
    - Fibroid degeneration ('red degeneration'):
        - inadequate blood supply to the fibroid causes haemorrhage and necrosis;
        - there is pain and uterine tenderness;
        - tends to occur during pregnancy.
    - Torsion of pedunculated fibroids.
    - Malignancy:
        - leiomyosarcoma;
        - rare;
        - more common in white than Afro-Caribbean women.
    - Complications in pregnancy can also occur, including:
        - premature labour;
        - malpresentation;
        - postpartum haemorrhage;
        - obstruction of labour.

13.5 BENIGN CONDITIONS OF THE CERVIX

CERVICAL ECTROPION

- This is a red ring visible on the ectocervix: the part of the cervix that is continuous with the vagina and covered in squamous epithelium.
- It is due to the presence of columnar epithelium, which is only one cell thick, less resistant and therefore more prone to bleeding.
- Ectropion tends to occur with increased oestrogen production: during puberty, pregnancy and with the combined pill. It is a normal finding.
- Occasionally it causes vaginal discharge, post-coital bleeding or contact bleeding, e.g. following a smear.

CERVICITIS

- Infection of the cervical epithelium.
- May be acute or chronic.
- Common causes include *Chlamydia*, gonococci and herpes.
- It is rare.

POLYPS

- Benign tumours of cervical epithelium.
- Most commonly arise at the endocervix.
- Often found incidentally at the time of routine cervical cytology.
- May cause inter-menstrual bleeding or post-coital bleeding.

Gynaecology

NABOTHIAN CYSTS

- Mucus-filled cysts that form on the surface of the ectocervix.
- They are formed by blockage of the glands of the columnar epithelium, owing to squamous cell metaplasia.
- They are physiological and usually asymptomatic, although they may occasionally cause a discharge.
- No action is necessary.

13.6 BENIGN CONDITIONS OF THE OVARIES

BENIGN OVARIAN CYSTS

- **Epidemiology**:
  - fourth most common cause of gynaecological admissions;
  - tend to occur in women of reproductive age.
- **Classification**:
  - see Table 13.2.

Table 13.2 Classification of ovarian cysts.

GROUP	CYST TYPE
Epithelial	Serous cystadenoma
	Mucinous cystadenoma
	Brenner tumour
Germ cell	Dermoid cysts
Sex cord tumours	Fibroma
	Granulosa
	Theca
Inflammatory	Endometriomas
Functional	Follicular
	Luteal

- **Epithelial tumours**:
  - Most common in women >40 years:
    - Serous cystadenoma:
      - ○ most common epithelial tumour;
      - ○ unilocular;
      - ○ approximately 30% are malignant.

- Mucinous cystadenoma:
  - can be very large and multiloculated;
  - less frequently malignant.
- Brenner tumours:
  - rare;
  - small and mostly benign.
- **Germ cell tumours**:
  - Dermoid cyst:
    - The most commonly occurring benign germ cell tumour.
    - Usually occur in women <30 years old.
    - Originate from all three germ cell layers and therefore often contain teeth and hair.
    - Usually asymptomatic but they can rupture or undergo torsion.
    - MRI is useful for diagnosis.
    - Treatment:
      - Cystectomy. The aim is to remove the cyst intact, preventing rupture into the peritoneal cavity. If the cyst is large, suspicious or technically thought to be too difficult to remove then an oophorectomy is performed.
      - Complete oophorectomy may be required if torsion occurs.
- **Sex cord tumours**:
  - These tumours secrete hormones (usually oestrogen) and therefore tend to present with symptoms related to the hormone produced.
  - Fibroma:
    - Most common type.
    - Small, solid tumours.
    - Associated with Meig's syndome (very rare):
      - pleural effusion, ascites and ovarian fibroma.
  - Granulosa cell tumours:
    - rare;
    - malignant but slow growing;
    - secrete oestrogens which may cause post-menopausal bleeding and even endometrial malignancy.
  - Thecomas:
    - very rare;
    - benign;
    - secrete oestrogens with similar affects to granulosa cell tumours.
- **Inflammatory cysts**:
  - Endometriomas ('chocolate cysts'):
    - arise as a complication of endometriosis (see Endometriosis);
    - consist of menstrual blood that accumulates in the ovary as a cyst;

Gynaecology

- these cysts can also occur elsewhere in the abdomen and pelvis;
- they have a characteristic 'ground-glass' appearance on ultrasound scan;
- rupture is very painful;
- laparoscopic ovarian cystectomy is required.

- **Functional cysts:**
  - Arise from follicles and corpora lutea: follicles which have ruptured to release an ovum.
  - Only occur in pre-menopausal women as they arise through the physiological process of folliculogenesis.
  - Usually asymptomatic but symptoms may occur owing to oestrogen secretion from the cysts.
  - Follicular cysts:
    - most common;
    - unilocular and up to 10 cm in diameter.
  - Corpus luteal cysts:
    - occur following ovulation;
    - tend to cause more symptoms;
    - if asymptomatic they can be observed using serial ultrasound scans.
  - Symptomatic cysts may require removal by laparoscopic cystectomy.

- **Clinical features:**
  - Presentation varies depending on size and type.
  - Often asymptomatic and a chance finding (e.g. on ultrasound) but symptoms may include:
    - bloating;
    - pain due to torsion, rupture or haemorrhage;
    - menstrual disturbance;
    - pressure effects on adjacent organs, e.g. urinary frequency.
  - On examination there may be a palpable abdominal mass, distension or ascites.

- **Investigations:**
  - Transvaginal ultrasound scan:
    - to assess the size, site and nature of the cyst.
  - CT or MRI.
  - Tumour markers:
    - poor sensitivity.
    - CA-125 may be elevated in epithelial ovarian cancer.
  - Risk of malignancy index (see Chapter 14, Gynaecological malignancies):
    - allows triage of women into those who are sufficiently low risk to allow conservative management and those who will require some form of intervention.

- **Management**:
  - depends on the nature of the cyst and any presenting symptoms;
  - differs depending on whether the woman is pre- or post-menopausal (see Table 13.3);
  - torsion and rupture warrant urgent surgery.

MICRO-facts

Complications of cysts
1. Rupture.
2. Torsion.
3. Haemorrhage into a cyst.
4. Malignant change.

Rupture, torsion and haemorrhage cause severe abdominal pain.

Table 13.3 Management of ovarian cysts in pre- and post-menopausal women.

	CYST FEATURES	MANAGEMENT
Pre-menopausal	<3 cm	Normal No further action required
	<5 cm Simple, asymptomatic	Reassure Re-scan in 3 months
	5–10 cm Simple, asymptomatic	Repeat ultrasound scan in 6 weeks
	5–10 cm Increasing in size or symptomatic	Diagnostic laparoscopy/laparotomy
Post-menopausal	Low risk of malignancy <5 cm Simple, unilateral	Repeat scan every 4 months (max. 12 months); if increasing in size or any suspicious features then patient will need laparoscopic oophorectomy or staging laparotomy
	Intermediate risk	Laparoscopic oophorectomy (if malignancy is revealed a full staging laparotomy is required)
	High risk	Full staging laparotomy

Gynaecology

13.7 BENIGN CONDITIONS OF THE VULVA

LICHEN SIMPLEX CHRONICUS

- Dry and scaly skin lesions on the labia majora that arise due to scratching.
- The vulva may become quite sore as a result.
- It is the end stage of an 'itch–scratch–itch' cycle.
- The itching causes thickening of the skin and increased skin markings. The skin may appear whitish and this is called lichenification.
- Treatment:
  - emollients and low-potency steroids.

LICHEN PLANUS

- Itchy, flat purple papules on the vulva.
- Loss of vulval architecture.
- Skin, hair, nails and mucous membranes (particularly oral mucosa) may be affected.
- Autoimmune condition:
  - check thyroid function.
- Treatment:
  - emollients and topical or (less commonly) systemic steroids.

LICHEN SCLEROSUS

- Inflammatory white papules on the skin of the vulva. These patches may unite, resulting in vulval skin that is thin, itchy and sore.
- Loss of vulval architecture:
  - fusion of the labia minora and majora.
- Most common in post-menopausal women.
- Unknown aetiology: possibly autoimmune.
- 2–5% of cases are associated with vulval carcinoma.
- Treatment:
  - emollients and potent steroids.

BARTHOLINITIS

- Bartholin's glands sit at the posterior aspect of the introitus and secrete lubricating mucus.
- If the glands become blocked a cyst may form:
  - this is typically unilateral and asymptomatic.
- Secondary infection results in abscess formation:
  - Common causative organisms are *Staphylococcus*, *Streptococcus*, *Escherichia coli* and gonorrhoea (rare).
  - The abscess is usually very tender.
  - Treatment includes:

- Antibiotics.
- Analgesia.
- Surgical drainage.
- Marsupialization:
    ○ creation of a new duct in order to prevent recurrence.

VAGINAL AND VULVAL INFECTION

- A number of infections may affect the vulva (see Chapter 19, Genital tract infections):
    - genital warts;
    - herpes simplex;
    - candidiasis;
    - syphilis.

MICRO-print

Discussion of the vulval pain syndromes is beyond the scope of this book. It is a diagnosis of exclusion commonly associated with a previous history of genital tract infection and psychosexual problems.

13.8 URINARY TRACT INFECTION

- **Definition**:
    - infection anywhere in the urinary tract from the kidneys to the bladder;
    - may be bacterial or fungal;
    - pyelonephritis is the term used to describe infection in the renal parenchyma;
    - cystitis refers to localized bladder infection.
- **Epidemiology**:
    - very common in women because of a shorter urethra;
    - 60% of women have had at least one urinary tract infection.
- **Pathophysiology**:
    - Transurethral ascent of micro-organisms from the perineum. The following factors increase the risk of cystitis:
        - urinary obstruction or stasis;
        - bladder stones;
        - catheters;
        - poor bladder emptying;
        - sexual intercourse: particularly with a new partner.

- **Aetiology**:
  - Causative organisms tend to originate from the patient's own bowel flora:
    - most commonly this is *E. coli;*
    - *Staphylococcus saprophyticus* is an important causative organism in young, sexually active women;
    - other common bacterial causes include *Proteus mirabilis* and *Klebsiella* spp.;
    - fungal infections are rare.
- **Clinical features of lower urinary tract infection**:
  - **History**:
    - Dysuria.
    - Urinary frequency.
    - Urgency.
    - Suprapubic pain.
    - Haematuria.
    - Offensive or cloudy urine.
  - **Examination**:
    - The following symptoms may be present:
      - ○ pyrexia: tends to occur in pyelonephritis;
      - ○ lower abdominal pain and tenderness;
      - ○ unilateral flank tenderness.

MICRO-facts

The symptoms of acute pyelonephritis are those of a lower urinary tract infection plus:

- unilateral flank and loin pain;
- fever;
- rigors.

- **Investigations**:
  - Urine dipstick:
    - positive for leucocytes, nitrites, blood and protein.
  - Urine microscopy, culture and sensitivity:
    - significant pyuria: $> 10^5$ pus cells per high-power field;
    - significant bacteriuria: $> 10^5$/mL pure growth of bacteria;
    - this also determines the sensitivity and resistance of the organism to various antibiotics.
  - Full blood count: neutrophilia.

- **Treatment**:
  - Advise increased oral fluid intake to help flush out the bacteria.
  - Analgesia.
  - 3–5 day course of antibiotics (consult local guidelines). Commonly:
    - trimethoprim;
    - nitrofurantoin;
    - amoxicillin;
    - co-amoxiclav.
  - Patients with acute pyelonephritis require hospital admission and treatment with intravenous antibiotics.
  - Repeat mid-stream specimen of urine 48 hours after finishing antibiotics to ensure adequate treatment.

MICRO-facts

In patients with a catheter, the urine dipstick is often positive. Treatment is only indicated if the patient is symptomatic.

---

14 Gynaecological malignancies

14.1 ENDOMETRIAL CARCINOMA

- **Epidemiology**:
    - most common genital tract malignancy;
    - fourth most common malignancy in women;
    - median age of diagnosis is 62 years.
- **Pathology**:
    - >90% are adenocarcinomas.
- **Aetiology**:
    - endometrial carcinoma results from the unopposed action of oestrogen on the uterus in the absence of progesterone, which has a protective effect.

> ## MICRO-facts
>
> The sole use of oestrogen therapy greatly increases the risk of developing endometrial cancer.
>
> The majority of endometrial cancer risk factors pertain to increased oestrogen exposure, whereas progesterone has a protective effect. As such the combined oral contraceptive pill and pregnancy have a protective effect on the endometrium.

- **Risk factors**:
    - Obesity.
    - Polycystic ovary syndrome.
    - Early menarche.
    - Late menopause.
    - Nulliparity.
    - Oestrogen-secreting ovarian tumours.
    - Tamoxifen:
        - acts as an oestrogen antagonist in the breast but an oestrogen agonist in the endometrium.

- **Clinical features**:
  - post-menopausal bleeding with/without discharge;
  - pre-menopausal women may notice a change to their usual cycle and experience irregular, inter-menstrual or heavier bleeding.

MICRO-facts

Post-menopausal bleeding is endometrial carcinoma until proven otherwise.

- **Screening**:
  - Endometrial carcinoma presents early; therefore, screening is not routine.
- **Investigations**:
  - Transvaginal ultrasound scan.
  - If the endometrium is >5 mm thick a pipelle biopsy is taken:
    - a pipelle is a type of curette;
    - it is passed through the cervical os into the endometrium and a sample of endometrial tissue is taken;
    - it can be performed in an outpatient setting.
  - Hysteroscopy and biopsy:
    - may be required if the woman is unable to tolerate a pipelle or the specimen is inadequate.
- **Staging**:
  - staged histologically using the FIGO (International Federation of Gynecology and Obstetrics) system.

MICRO-print

A summary of the FIGO staging system:

Stage I Confined to the uterus.
Stage II Includes the cervix but it has not extended outside the uterus.
Stage III Extends out through the uterus but remains in the pelvis.
Stage IV Includes bladder, bowel or distant metastases.

MICRO-reference

http://www.figo.org/publications/staging_classifications

- **Treatment**:
  - Laparotomy (if surgically fit) with total abdominal hysterectomy (TAH) and bilateral salpingo-oophorectomy (BSO) with/without lymphadenectomy.
  - Adjuvant radiotherapy:
    - external beam pelvic radiation and vault brachytherapy.
  - Chemotherapy:
    - usually in a trial setting or if an unusual histological type.
- **Prognosis**:
  - depends on the grade, stage and type of tumour;
  - overall, 75% 5 year survival.

MICRO-reference

National Institute for Health and Clinical Excellence. Laparoscopic hysterectomy (including laparoscopic total hysterectomy and laparoscopically assisted vaginal hysterectomy) for endometrial cancer. London, UK: NICE, 2008. Available at http://www.nice.org.uk/nicemedia/live/12355/50832/50832.pdf

---

14.2 OVARIAN CARCINOMA

- **Epidemiology**:
  - causes the most gynaecological cancer deaths;
  - typically occurs in women between 60 and 70 years old;
  - more common in developed nations.

MICRO-reference

National Institute for Health and Clinical Excellence. Ovarian cancer: the recognition and initial management of ovarian cancer. London, UK: NICE, 2011. Available at http://www.nice.org.uk/nicemedia/live/13464/54194/54194.pdf

---

- **Pathology**:
  - Primary tumours:
    - may be epithelial, germ cell or sex cord in origin;
    - epithelial tumours account for 90% of ovarian cancers;
    - germ cell tumours tend to occur in younger women.
  - Secondary tumours:
    - account for 6% of ovarian tumours;
    - may arise from breast, bowel, stomach or thyroid.

- **Aetiology**:
  - An increased number of ovulations predisposes to malignant transformation.
  - Risk factors include:
    - early menarche;
    - late menopause;
    - nulliparity.
  - Protective factors include:
    - lactation;
    - multiparity;
    - the combined oral contraceptive pill.
  - A small number of cases are familial: associated with *BRCA1* and *BRCA2* mutations and hereditary non-polyposis colorectal cancer.
- **Clinical features**:
  - Most are not diagnosed until the disease is advanced, since:
    - Silent in early stages.
    - Non-specific abdominal symptoms:
      - ○ pain, discomfort, bloating, flatulence and increasing abdominal girth.
  - 75% present at stages 3 or 4 (see later) with abdominal distension, mass or pain.
- **Screening**:
  - not routine at present;
  - currently being evaluated by the United Kingdom Collaborative Trial on Ovarian Cancer Screening.
- **Investigations**:
  - To help establish diagnosis and stage:
    - Ultrasound scan of the abdomen and pelvis.
    - Tumour markers CA-125 and CA-19-9 may be elevated.
    - If an ovarian cancer is suspected the risk of malignancy index (RMI) should be used to predict whether the mass is malignant or not:
      - ○ ultrasound features, CA-125 and menopausal status are used to calculate the score;
      - ○ RMI = menopausal status × ultrasound features × CA-125.
    - Metastatic spread can be assessed with a CT scan of the abdomen, pelvis and chest.
  - To assess fitness for surgery:
    - Full blood count, urea and electrolytes and liver function tests.
- **Staging**:
  - determined following surgery;
  - based on the FIGO classification.

Gynaecology

MICRO-print

The FIGO staging system is summarized below:

- **Stage I**: tumour confined to the ovaries.
  - Ia: confined to one ovary, capsule intact, no ascites.
  - Ib: limited to both ovaries, capsules intact, no ascites.
  - Ic: limited to one or both ovaries, but capsule ruptured, tumour present on surface of ovary, malignant ascites of positive peritoneal washings.
- **Stage II**: tumour involves one or both ovaries and has extended into the pelvis.
  - IIa: extension and/or metastases to uterus or fallopian tubes.
  - IIb: extension to other pelvic organs.
  - IIc: IIa/IIb with malignant ascites or positive peritoneal washings.
- **Stage III**: involves the ovaries with metastases beyond the pelvis into the abdomen.
  - IIIa: microscopic peritoneal metastasis.
  - IIIb: macroscopic peritoneal metastasis <2 cm in diameter.
  - IIIc: macroscopic peritoneal metastasis >2 cm in diameter and/ or regional lymph node metastasis.
- **Stage IV**: distant metastases beyond the abdomen or involving the liver parenchyma.

MICRO-reference

http://www.figo.org/publications/staging_classifications

- **Treatment**:
  - 'Staging' laparotomy, consisting of:
    - TAH and BSO;
    - infracolic omentectomy;
    - para-aortic node dissection;
    - peritoneal washings for cytology;
    - if ascites is present the fluid is sent for cytology;
    - examination of all intra-abdominal peritoneal surfaces to assess for metastatic spread.
  - If the tumour has metastasized, it will require surgical debulking and chemotherapy.
- **Prognosis**:
  - overall 5 year survival rate <35%;
  - however, survival rates have increased twofold over the last 30 years owing to developments in chemotherapy and surgical practice.

MICRO-facts

It is important that all gynaecological cancer cases are discussed at a multidisciplinary team meeting in order to decide on the most appropriate treatment.

MICRO-reference

National Institute for Health and Clinical Excellence. Ovarian cancer: the recognition and initial management of ovarian cancer. London, UK: NICE, 2011. Available at http://www.nice.org.uk/nicemedia/live/13464/54194/54194.pdf

MICRO-case

A 62-year-old woman presented to her GP with a 6 month history of abdominal discomfort and bloating. She had made several trips to the GP in the past and her symptoms had been attributed to irritable bowel syndrome. However, her symptoms were getting progressively worse and she was feeling very anxious.

Other than hypertension, which was well controlled with amlodipine, she had no other medical problems.

On examination of the abdomen there was ascites but no palpable masses. Vaginal examination revealed a fixed right-sided pelvic mass.

The GP did a series of blood tests, which showed the following:

- CA-125   567 (<30)
- Haemoglobin   10.4 (11.5–16.5)
- White cell count   6 (4–11)
- Platelets   267 (150 – 450)

The patient was referred urgently to gynaecology. An ultrasound scan confirmed the presence of ascites and a 6 cm right-sided ovarian mass strongly suggestive of an ovarian malignancy. The patient was deemed medically fit for surgery and underwent a 'staging' laparotomy. Histology confirmed the diagnosis of ovarian cancer. The tumour had metastasized to the bowel serosa and liver but CT of the abdomen, thorax and pelvis revealed no extra-abdominal involvement. It was confirmed as a stage III ovarian carcinoma. The patient received chemotherapy because of the late stage.

Key points:

- Most women with ovarian cancer have non-specific symptoms and it is for this reason that it tends to present with late stage disease.
- Ovarian cancer is rare in young women.
- Surgery is necessary for diagnosis, staging and treatment provided the patient is medically fit for anaesthetic.
- Survival remains poor, largely because of the late presentation.

Gynaecology

14.3 CERVICAL INTRA-EPITHELIAL NEOPLASIA

- **Definition**:
  - histological abnormality of the cervix in which abnormal epithelial cells are present in the squamous epithelium.
- **Classification**:
  - see Table 14.1.

Table 14.1 Classification of cervical intra-epithelial neoplasia (CIN).

GRADE	DEFINITION	MANAGEMENT
Borderline		Repeat smear 6 months later. Colposcopy required after three borderline smears
CIN I: mild dyskaryosis	Atypical cells in lower third of epithelium	Colposcopy (one repeat test is acceptable)
CIN II: moderate dyskaryosis	Atypical cells in lower two-thirds of epithelium	Colposcopy
CIN III: severe dyskaryosis	Atypical cells throughout the epithelium (carcinoma *in situ*)	Colposcopy
Glandular neoplasia	Atypical glandular cells in the cervical canal	Urgent colposcopy

> **MICRO-reference**
> http://www.cks.nhs.uk/cervical_screening/management/scenario_when_to_offer_cervical_screening/unscheduled_cervical_screening/basis_for_recommendation#-451679.

- **Epidemiology and aetiology**:
  - In 99.7% of cases, human papillomavirus (HPV) is responsible for the neoplastic changes (CIN) that occur within cervical cells. These may subsequently become malignant.
  - HPV types 16 and 18 are associated with the development of CIN:
    - HPV is a sexually transmitted infection; the risk of infection increases the more sexual partners a person has had, particularly at a young age;

- the majority of women will clear the virus; a minority retain oncogenic HPV that can lead to the development of CIN.
- Other associated factors include:
  - smoking;
  - immunocompromise, e.g. human immunodeficiency virus;
  - genital warts;
  - high-risk male partner.
- **Pathophysiology**:
  - During puberty, oestrogens and a lower vaginal pH cause the columnar epithelium lining the endocervix to undergo metaplasia to squamous epithelium.
  - The area where metaplasia occurs is called the 'transformation zone'.
  - Cells in the transformation zone are subsequently more prone to CIN.

MICRO-facts

A vaccine has been developed against human papillomavirus (HPV) types 6, 11, 16 and 18 and is licensed for 9–35-year-olds. The UK vaccination programme is targeted at 12–13-year-old girls to prevent HPV infection types 16 and 18. The aim is for girls to be vaccinated before becoming sexually active, in order to reduce the number of cases of CIN and subsequently the number of cases of cervical cancer.

For more information, go to the national vaccination programme website (http://www.cdc.gov/vaccines/).

- **Clinical features**:
  - usually asymptomatic; identified by cervical screening;
  - not visible on the cervix.
- **Investigations**:
  - **Cervical screening**:
    - Cervical smears are performed on women >25 years every 3 years until the age of 50. Between the ages of 50 and 64, smears are 5 yearly provided that results are normal.
    - Analysis by liquid-based cytology is the current technology used:
      - A plastic broom is swept around the external cervical os in order to remove a layer of cells, which are then placed in a buffer solution and processed before being examined under a microscope.
    - Identifies dyskaryosis, not histological abnormalities.
    - See Table 14.1.

> ## MICRO-facts
>
> Dyskaryosis is a term used to describe the cellular (not the histological) appearance of the superficial cells sampled following a cervical smear. It does not mean that cervical intra-epithelial neoplasia (CIN) is present, just that if a biopsy were to be performed it may be likely to show that particular stage of CIN.

- **Colposcopy**:
  - Performed if a cervical smear is severely or persistently abnormal.
  - Enables visualization of the cervix with bright light and magnification.
  - The cervix is stained with 5% acetic acid, highlighting the characteristics of the different CIN grades.
  - The colposcopist makes an assessment as to whether the CIN is low or high grade:
    - ○ high-grade CIN is treated at the time in the clinic;
    - ○ low-grade CIN can be monitored with cytology 6 months later with/without colposcopy; if the abnormal area is large or the patient is anxious, treatment may be performed;
    - ○ biopsies of abnormal areas should be taken.

> ## MICRO-print
> ### Shiller's test
>
> - Lugol's iodine can also be used to identify abnormalities on the cervix.
> - Normal squamous epithelium contains glycogen, which stains brown/black.
> - Pre-cancerous and cancerous lesions do not contain glycogen and so do not take up the iodine. They appear as yellow areas.
> - Some colposcopists use iodine and acetic acid; others use only acetic acid.

- **Treatment**:
  - The aim is to treat pre-cancer before it progresses to invasion.
  - CIN I can be treated or observed:
    - as mentioned above the smear is repeated in 6 months' time.
  - CIN II and III are treated by large loop excision of the transformation zone.

MICRO-print
Cervical glandular intra-epithelial neoplasia

- Rare.
- Less well detected on smear testing than squamous lesions, and difficult to assess on colposcopy as it tends to arise in the cervical canal.
- Treatment is with surgical excision under general anaesthetic.
- Hysterectomy should be considered if fertility is no longer required or the margins are not clear, because of the inaccuracy of follow-up.

MICRO-reference
The British Society for Colposcopy and Cervical Pathology. Available at http://www.bsccp.org.uk/index.asp?PageID = 1
NHS Cervical Cancer Screening Programme. Available at http://www.cancerscreening.nhs.uk/cervical/index.html

14.4 CERVICAL CANCER

- **Epidemiology**:
  - becoming less common in the UK as a result of the screening programme;
  - third most common gynaecological malignancy.
- **Pathology**:
  - 90% are squamous cell carcinoma.
- **Aetiology**:
  - see Cervical intra-epithelial neoplasia.
- **Risk factors**:
  - HPV: see before;
  - smoking;
  - combined oral contraceptive pill;
  - immunosuppression.
- **Clinical features**:
  - post-coital bleeding;
  - inter-menstrual bleeding;
  - post-menopausal bleeding;
  - bloodstained, offensive smelling vaginal discharge;
  - on examination the cervix may appear normal in early disease; later it may be ulcerated or replaced by an irregular mass.

Gynaecology

- **Screening**:
  - see above;
  - if the woman has cancer then the screening programme has failed that woman.
- **Investigations**:
  - colposcopy;
  - cervical biopsy;
  - full blood count, urea and electrolytes and liver function tests in order to assess fitness for surgery;
  - MRI pelvis: for staging and to help plan treatment.
- **Staging**:
  - determined clinically following an examination an under an anaesthetic with/without cystoscopy and sigmoidoscopy.

MICRO-print

The FIGO staging system is summarized below:

- **Stage I**: confined to the cervix.
  - Ia: invasive cancer only identified microscopically.
  - Ia1: invasion ≤3 mm in depth and diameter ≤7 mm.
  - Ia2: invasion >3–5 mm in depth and >7 mm diameter.
  - Ib: clinical lesions confined to the cervix or pre-clinical lesions greater than stage Ia.
  - Ib1: clinical lesions no greater than 4 cm in size.
  - Ib2: clinical lesions greater than 4 cm in size.
- **Stage II**: extends beyond the cervix but not into the pelvic wall (involves the vagina but not the lower third).
  - IIa: up to the upper two-thirds of the vagina involved.
  - IIb: infiltration of the parametrium.
- **Stage III**: extends into the pelvic side-wall and to the lower third of the vagina.
  - IIIa: lower third of the vagina involved.
  - IIIb: extension into the pelvic side-wall or hydronephrosis or non-functioning kidney.
- **Stage IV**: includes bladder and/or rectum and distant organs.
  - IVa: spread to adjacent pelvic organs.
  - IVb: spread to distant organs.

MICRO-reference

http://www.figo.org/publications/staging_classifications

- **Treatment**:
  - depends on clinical stage;
  - microinvasion (stage Ia) requires a cone biopsy or simple hysterectomy;
  - stages Ib and IIa are treated with hysterectomy with/without radiotherapy and chemotherapy;
  - stages IIb, III and IV are treated with radiotherapy and chemotherapy without surgery.
- **Prognosis**:
  - depends on lymph node involvement, clinical stage and histological grade;
  - overall 65% 5 year survival.

14.5 VULVAL INTRA-EPITHELIAL NEOPLASIA

- **Definition**:
  - histological abnormality of the vulva in which abnormal cells are present in the vulval epithelium.
- **Classification**:
  - similar classification system to CIN (see Cervical intra-epithelial neoplasia);
  - vulval intra-epithelial neoplasia (VIN) I–III where VIN III is carcinoma *in situ*.
- **Pathophysiology**:
  - There are two main causes of VIN:
    - HPV: tends to be associated with the development of VIN in women under the age of 45;
    - lichen sclerosis: predominantly associated with VIN in older women.
  - In 5–10% of cases, VIN progresses to vulval carcinoma.
- **Clinical features**:
  - pruritus or pain;
  - white papular lesions;
  - often asymptomatic; may be an incidental finding at colposcopy.
- **Investigations**:
  - vulvoscopy;
  - biopsy.
- **Treatment**:
  - local excision: usually only of symptomatic areas owing to high recurrence rates;
  - imiquimod (topical chemotherapy);
  - the main aim is to alleviate symptoms and be alert for progression to cancer by serial examination and biopsy.

14.6 VULVAL CARCINOMA

- **Epidemiology**:
    - vulval carcinoma is rare and accounts for less than 6% of gynaecological malignancies;
    - it is most common in women over the age of 65.
- **Pathophysiology**:
    - over 90% of vulval carcinomas originate from squamous cells;
    - many arise from the development and progression of VIN; however, they can arise *de novo*;
    - they are skin tumours of the vulva, and so malignant melanoma and basal cell carcinoma can also occur.

MICRO-reference

http://cancerhelp.cancerresearchuk.org/type/vulval-cancer/about/risks-and-causes-of-vulval-cancer#common

---

- **Clinical features**:
    - History:
        - pruritus;
        - bleeding;
        - discharge;
        - pain.
    - Examination:
        - ulcer;
        - mass;
        - most commonly found on the labia majora and clitoris.
- **Investigations**:
    - biopsy to establish the diagnosis.
- **Staging**:
    - based on surgery and histology;
    - follows the FIGO guidelines.

MICRO-print

The FIGO staging system is summarized as:

Stage I Lesions confined to the vulva or perineum ≤2 cm in size.
Stage II Lesions confined to the vulva and/or perineum >2 cm in size.
Stage III Tumour has spread beyond the vulva and perineum to the urethra, vagina or anus and/or nodes are affected unilaterally.
Stage IV Bilateral lymph node involvement and/or distant metastases.

MICRO-reference
http://www.figo.org/publications/staging_classifications

- **Treatment**:
    - wide local excision for stage I disease with minimal stromal invasion;
    - vulvectomy and groin lymphadenectomy for the other stages;
    - radiotherapy is an alternative to surgery but has higher recurrence rates; it may also be used after surgery to reduce the risk of local recurrence.
- **Prognosis**:
    - >90% 5 year survival for stage I disease;
    - may be as low as 10% 5 year survival for stage IV disease;
    - melanomas usually have a poor prognosis.

MICRO-reference
http://www.cancer.gov – for all gynaecological cancers.

Gynaecology

15 Urogynaecology

15.1 STRESS URINARY INCONTINENCE

- **Definition**:
    - the involuntary leakage of urine that occurs when bladder pressure exceeds maximum urethral pressure, in the absence of a detrusor contraction.

MICRO-reference

Impey L. Disorders of the urinary tract. In: Impey L (ed.). Obstetrics and gynaecology, 2nd edn. Oxford, UK: Wiley-Blackwell, 2004, pp. 51–8.

- **Epidemiology**:
    - The prevalence of stress urinary incontinence (SUI) and overactive bladder is now approximately equal:
        - it tends to increase up to the age of 50, reaches a plateau at age 50–70 and steadily increases with age thereafter.

Table 15.1 Terminology of urinary symptoms.

TERM	DEFINITION
Increased frequency	The patient feels they void too often
Nocturia	Micturition more than once during the night
Urgency	A sudden and compelling desire to void
Urge urinary incontinence	Incontinence accompanied, or preceded, by urgency
Stress urinary incontinence	Incontinence when intra-abdominal pressure increases, e.g. on coughing

Data from International Urogynecological Association/International Continence Society. Joint report on the terminology for female pelvic floor dysfunction. Bristol, UK: ICS, 2009. Available at http://www.icsoffice.org/Documents/Documents.aspx?DocumentID=611

MICRO-reference
International Urogynecological Association/International Continence Society. Joint report on the terminology for female pelvic floor dysfunction. Bristol, UK: ICS, 2009. Available at http://www.icsoffice.org/Documents/Documents.aspx?DocumentID =611

- **Risk factors**:
    - Increasing age (post-menopausal).
    - Pregnancy:
        - resolves spontaneously after birth in most women.
    - Obstetric factors:
        - vaginal delivery;
        - instrumental delivery;
        - prolonged labour.
    - Obesity.
    - Parity.
- **Pathophysiology**:
    - Weakened bladder supports cause the bladder neck to slip below the pelvic floor.
    - When the intra-abdominal pressure increases (e.g. when coughing) the bladder is compressed but the bladder neck is not.
    - This results in a higher pressure in the bladder than in the bladder neck.
    - Incontinence results if the urethra and pelvic floor muscles cannot compensate for this pressure increase.
- **Clinical features**:
    - History:
        - Stress incontinence: this is the usual symptom.
        - Frequency.
        - Urgency or urge incontinence may also occur.
        - Faecal incontinence may occur as a result of injury at childbirth.
        - Check fluid intake and types:
            - ○ tea, coffee and alcohol all have a diuretic effect.
        - Drug history, e.g. diuretics.

MICRO-facts

When taking a history from a patient with urinary incontinence it is essential to assess the degree to which the patient's life has been disrupted. Asking the woman how many times a day she has to change her pad can be a useful indicator of the severity of the incontinence.

Gynaecology

- Examination:
  - Stress incontinence may be demonstrated when the patient coughs.
  - Bimanual:
    ○ assess the strength of the pelvic floor muscles by asking the woman to squeeze.
  - Speculum:
    ○ may reveal a cystourethrocele (see Uterovaginal prolapse).
  - Abdomen:
    ○ palpation of the abdomen to assess for masses.

MICRO-facts

Stress urinary incontinence and overactive bladder may both present with stress incontinence. The management of these conditions is very different; therefore, cystometry is essential in order to exclude overactive bladder.

- **Investigations**:
  - Urine culture:
    - To exclude infection.
  - Blood sugar:
    - To exclude diabetes if experiencing urinary frequency.
  - Cystometry:
    - Indication:
      ○ to differentiate between SUI and overactive bladder.
    - Procedure:
      ○ transducers are placed in the rectum and bladder in order to measure intra-abdominal and intra-vesical pressure respectively;
      ○ the intra-vesical transducer is usually attached to the catheter that is used to fill the bladder;
      ○ detrusor pressure = bladder pressure – abdominal pressure;
      ○ the detrusor pressure should not increase with an increase in intra-abdominal pressure, on filling or provocation.
    - Demonstrates the following:
      ○ leakage of urine in the absence of a detrusor contraction (see Table 15.2).
- **Treatment**:
  - Lifestyle measures:
    - Weight loss.
    - Smoking cessation.
    - Avoid tea, coffee and alcohol.
    - Restriction of daily fluid intake.

Table 15.2 Cystometry interpretation.

	NORMAL BLADDER	STRESS URINARY INCONTINENCE	OVERACTIVE BLADDER
Increased detrusor contractions on bladder filling	No	No	Yes
Detrusor contraction on coughing	No	No	No (contraction occurs following a cough)
Urine flow with cough	No	Yes	No

Data from Impey L. Disorders of the urinary tract. In: Impey L (ed.). Obstetrics and gynaecology, 2nd edn. Oxford, UK: Wiley-Blackwell, 2004, pp. 51–8.

- Conservative:
  - The aim is to strengthen the pelvic floor. This can be achieved by physiotherapy-supervised pelvic floor muscle training:
    - 'vaginal cones';
    - these are placed into the vagina and held by voluntary muscle contraction;
    - increasingly large sizes are used as muscle strength increases.
  - Duloxetine, a selective serotonin reuptake inhibitor, may be offered as a second-line agent in women who do not wish to undergo surgery.

MICRO-facts

Pelvic floor muscle training is the first-line treatment and should be performed for 3 months before considering surgery.

- Surgical:
  - Tension-free vaginal tape (TVT):
    - less invasive than colposuspension (see below);
    - a polypropylene mesh is used to elevate the mid-urethra;
    - may be performed under a spinal or local anaesthetic;
    - shorter hospital stay.
  - Transobturator tape (TVT-O):
    - a newer type of surgical treatment, which works in the same way as the traditional TVT but is fitted in a slightly different way;
    - this method does not go near to the bladder and so the risk of bladder damage is less (see Complications).

Gynaecology

- Burch colposuspension:
  - previously the gold standard, but has now been replaced by the TVT;
  - it involves raising the vaginal wall from either side of the bladder neck up to the iliopectineal ligament using two non-absorbable sutures.
- Complications of surgery:
  - The following complications can occur with TVT and celposuspension but are less common with the TVT:
    ○ bleeding;
    ○ urinary tract infection;
    ○ urinary retention;
    ○ *de novo* detrusor overactivity.

MICRO-reference

Clinical Knowledge Summaries. Management of stress urinary incontinence symptoms. Available at http://www.cks.nhs.uk/incontinence_urinary_in_women/management/detailed_answers/secondary_care_treatments_for_urgency_incontinence#-368673

National Institute of Clinical Excellence. Urinary Incontinence. London, UK: NICE 2006. Available at: http://guidance.nice.org.uk/CG40/NICEGuidance/pdf/English

---

15.2 OVERACTIVE BLADDER

- **Definition**:
  - uninhibited detrusor contractions that can result in involuntary loss of urine.
- **Epidemiology**:
  - see Stress urinary incontinence.
- **Risk factors**:
  - idiopathic;
  - multiple sclerosis;
  - surgical treatment for stress urinary incontinence may cause bladder neck obstruction in some cases, resulting in an overactive bladder.
- **Pathophysiology**:
  - detrusor muscle contraction occurs, causing urgency;
  - if this contraction is strong enough, bladder pressure exceeds urethral pressure;
  - there is involuntary voiding of urine; this is known as urge incontinence.

- **Clinical features**:
  - History:
    - urgency;
    - urge incontinence;
    - frequency;
    - nocturia;
    - stress incontinence;
    - childhood enuresis;
    - faecal urgency.
  - Examination:
    - usually normal.
- **Investigations**:
  - Urinary diary:
    - a record of the patient's fluid intake and output.
  - Cystometry (see before):
    - on bladder filling this will demonstrate spontaneous or provoked detrusor contractions which the woman cannot suppress (see Table 15.2).
- **Treatment**: conservative:

> **MICRO-facts**
>
> It is essential to manage any underlying/contributing disease effectively, e.g. urinary tract infection, multiple sclerosis and diabetes mellitus.

- Lifestyle factors:
  - As for Stress urinary incontinence.
- Bladder drill:
  - This is the first-line treatment and should be undertaken for 6 weeks under the instruction of trained physiotherapists.
  - The aim is to re-train the bladder by timed voiding.
  - Rather than voiding at first desire, the patient voids at specified times. The interval between voids is gradually increased until a desired interval is reached.
- Pharmacological:
  - Anti-muscarinic drugs, e.g. tolterodine and oxybutynin:
    - mainstay of treatment for overactive bladder;
    - side-effects include: dry mouth, blurred vision, tachycardia and constipation;
    - tolterodine and oxybutynin are equally effective; however, the side-effect profile of tolterodine is slightly better.

Gynaecology

- Desmopressin:
  - ○ synthetic anti-diuretic hormone; unlicensed use;
  - ○ used to manage nocturnal polyuria in women.

- **Treatment**: non-conservative options:
  - Sacral nerve stimulation.
  - Augmentation cystoplasty:
    - The bladder is split in half and a segment of ileum is used to fill in the defect.
    - This disrupts the bladder contractions but usually results in the woman having to self-catheterize.
  - Urinary diversion:
    - ○ only considered if the above two measures fail.
  - Cystodistension:
    - while under a general anaesthetic, the patient is catheterized and approximately 500 mL of saline is instilled into the bladder;
    - the fluid is left in the bladder for approximately 10 minutes and then drained off;
    - it is not commonly used.
  - Botulinum toxin:
    - botulinum toxin A is injected into the bladder wall under cystoscopic control;
    - causes temporary paralysis of the detrusor muscle;
    - only suitable for women who have not responded to conservative measures and are prepared to self-catheterize;
    - there is a lack of long-term data.

MICRO-print

Approximately 10% of urinary incontinence is due to mixed urinary incontinence. It is a combination of stress urinary incontinence and overactive bladder, diagnosed by cystometry.

MICRO-reference

Clinical Knowledge Summaries. Secondary care treatments for urgency incontinence. Available at http://www.cks.nhs.uk/incontinence_urinary_in_women/management/detailed_answers/secondary_care_treatments_for_urgency_incontinence

National Institute of Clinical Excellence. Urinary Incontinence. London, UK: NICE 2006. Available at: http://guidance.nice.org.uk/CG40/NICEGuidance/pdf/English

15.3 UTEROVAGINAL PROLAPSE

- **Definition**:
    - the protrusion of the uterus and/or vaginal walls into the vagina.
- **Different types of uterovaginal prolapse**:
    - see Table 15.3.

Table 15.3 Different prolapse definitions.

TYPE OF PROLAPSE	DEFINITION
Anterior vaginal wall prolapse	
Cystocele	Descent of the bladder
Urethrocele	Descent of the urethra
Cystourethrocele	Descent of the bladder and urethra
Posterior vaginal wall prolapse	
Rectotocele	Descent of the rectum
Enterocele	Descent of the small bowel
Uterus/vaginal vault prolapse	
Uterus prolapse	Descent of the uterus
Vaginal vault prolapse (post-hysterectomy)	The vaginal vault (the apex of the vagina where the uterus used to be) can prolapse

MICRO-facts
Both anterior and posterior vaginal wall prolapses can be thought of as hernias.

MICRO-facts
Different definitions exist for the grading of uterus prolapses. The grading system in Table 15.4 is just one version. As a result, clinical examination is vital in prolapse assessment. To avoid any confusion, it is best to record what is seen during examination rather than use a grading system.

- **Epidemiology**:
    - affects 12–30% of parous women.
- **Aetiology**:
    - Childbirth:
        - vaginal delivery.
    - Ageing:
        - oestrogen deficiency causing atrophy of connective tissues.

Gynaecology

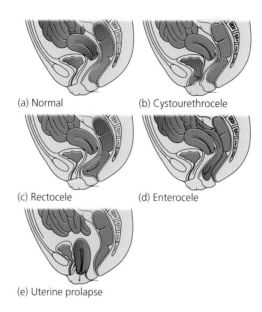

(a) Normal   (b) Cystourethrocele

(c) Rectocele   (d) Enterocele

(e) Uterine prolapse

Fig. 15.1 (a) Relationship of normal bladder, uterus and bowel. The different types of prolapse include: (b) cystourethrocele; (c) rectocele; (d) enterocele; and (e) uterine prolapse.

Table 15.4 Grading system for uterine prolapse.

GRADING	EXTENT OF DESCENT
First degree	Descent of cervix to introitus
Second degree	Descent of cervix (but not whole uterus) through the introitus
Third degree (procidentia)	Descent of cervix and whole uterus through the introitus

- Obesity.
- Raised intra-abdominal pressure:
  - chronic cough.
- Iatrogenic:
  - poorly supported vaginal vault post-hysterectomy.
- Congenital:
  - familial weakness of connective tissue supporting pelvic structures.

> **MICRO-print**
> **Pelvic supports**
>
> - **Transverse cervical ligaments**: attach uterus to pelvic walls.
> - **Uterosacral ligament**: attaches uterus to sacrum.
> - **Levator ani muscle**: forms the pelvis floor and suspends the vagina, urethra and rectum.
>
> Weakness of **transverse cervical and uterosacral** ligaments will result in prolapse of the uterus.
>
> Weakness of the **levator ani muscle** leads to prolapse of vaginal walls, urethra or rectum.

- **Clinical features**:
    - Asymptomatic.
    - Non-specific:
        - feeling of a lump;
        - discomfort;
        - backache.
    - Cystocele/urethrocystocele:
        - urinary frequency;
        - incomplete emptying;
        - stress incontinence.

> **MICRO-facts**
> Vaginal cysts and large uterine polyps may present similarly to prolapses.

    - Rectocele:
        - difficulty defaecating.
- **Investigations**:
    - no essential tests needed;
    - a pelvic ultrasound can be useful to exclude pelvic masses;
    - consider cystometry and cystoscopy if there are urinary symptoms.
- **Management**:
    - Conservative:
        - Weight reduction.
        - Physiotherapy to strengthen pelvic floor muscles.
        - Pessaries:
            - made from silicone;
            - inserted into the vagina and act like an artificial pelvic floor;
            - changed around every 4 months;

Gynaecology

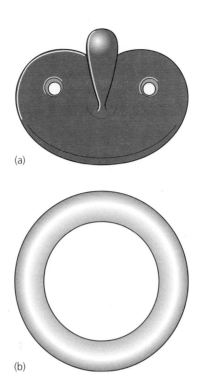

(a)

(b)

Fig. 15.2 (a) Shelf pessary and (b) ring pessary.

    ○ can cause vaginal ulceration in post-menopausal women; can give topical oestrogen or hormone replacement therapy on an intermittent basis as prevention;
    ○ there are two main types: ring pessary or shelf pessary (see Fig. 15.2);
    ○ shelf pessaries are usually used for vault prolapses.
- Surgery:
  – Anterior vaginal wall prolapses:
    ○ anterior repair: anterior vaginal wall is incised, fascia defect is repaired and any excess vaginal epithelium is excised.
  – Posterior vaginal wall prolapses.
    ○ posterior repair: posterior vaginal wall is incised, fascia defect is repaired and any excess vaginal epithelium is excised.
  – Uterine prolapse:
    ○ hysterectomy (if family complete).
  – Vaginal vault prolapse:
    ○ sacrospinous colpopexy (vaginally): attaching the vaginal vault to the sacrospinous ligament;
    ○ sacrocolpopexy (open or laparoscopic): attaching the vaginal vault to the sacrum.

MICRO-print
Meshes
There are many meshes that can be used by experts as second- or third-line treatments for uterovaginal prolapses. However, detailed information about these operations is beyond the scope of this text.

MICRO-case
A 76-year-old woman presented to her GP and complained of a discomfort 'down below'. She was a smoker and had chronic obstructive pulmonary disease (COPD) and hypertension. Her body mass index was 36. On further questioning, she described a feeling of there being a lump in her vagina. On examination, her cervix had descended into the vagina. The GP referred the patient to see a specialist in urogynaecology.

The urogynaecologist identified a first-degree uterus prolapse (descent of the cervix to the introitus). The patient was advised to lose some weight, and supervised physiotherapy to strengthen the pelvic floor muscles was suggested. The patient was happy to give this a try.

Three months later, the patient returned for her follow-up appointment. Her symptoms had improved slightly but were still bothersome. The patient was not keen for any surgery but wanted to know if anything else could be done. The urogynaecologist inserted a shelf pessary and prescribed some topical oestrogen cream. This controlled the prolapse and the patient continued to have this changed every 4 months.

Key points:

- Risk factors for a uterovaginal prolapse include obesity and causes of raised intra-abdominal pressure (chronic cough in COPD in this case).
- Always start with conservative management: it may be all that is required.

16 Disorders of early pregnancy

16.1 ECTOPIC PREGNANCY

- **Definition**:
  - implantation of the embryo outside of the uterus.
- **Epidemiology**:
  - rising incidence;
  - occurs in approximately 11:1000 pregnancies.
- **Pathophysiology**:
  - ectopic pregnancies most commonly occur in the fallopian tube;
  - the fallopian tube is unable to sustain trophoblastic invasion, resulting in bleeding into the lumen or rupture of the tube.
- **Risk factors**:
  - Anything which causes damage to the fallopian tube:
    - previous ectopic pregnancy;
    - pelvic inflammatory disease;
    - assisted conception;
    - pelvic surgery.
  - History of subfertility.
  - Progesterone-only pill.
  - Increasing age.
- **Clinical features**:
  - History:
    - Typically presents between 5 and 8 weeks' gestation.
    - Lower abdominal pain, typically colicky.
    - Sexually active.
    - Possibly a missed period, although the woman may not know that she is pregnant.
    - Vaginal bleeding:
      - ○ may be severe if the ectopic has ruptured;
      - ○ most bleeding occurs into the pelvic cavity; therefore, vaginal bleeding may be deceptively minimal.

- Less commonly, syncope (owing to blood loss), diarrhoea and vomiting may occur.
- May also be asymptomatic and an incidental finding on an early pregnancy scan.
  - Examination:
    - Signs of blood loss:
      ○ tachycardia.
      ○ hypotension and collapse – in severe cases.
    - Abdominal tenderness:
      ○ there may also be rebound tenderness and signs of peritonism if the ectopic has ruptured.
    - On pelvic examination:
      ○ cervical excitation may occur; this is pain on movement of the cervix;
      ○ unilateral adnexal tenderness may occur.
- **Investigations::**
  - Pregnancy test:
    - Almost always positive.

MICRO-facts

In any woman with a positive pregnancy test presenting with abdominal pain or vaginal bleeding the diagnosis is ectopic pregnancy until proven otherwise.

- Transvaginal ultrasound scan (TVS):
  - Can an intra-uterine gestational sac be visualized?
  - If the uterus is empty or the scan is inconclusive, human chorionic gonadotrophin (β-hCG) levels should be measured provided the woman is haemodynamically stable.
  - 15–50% of scans will be inconclusive.
- Quantitative measurement of β-hCG:
  - Two serum β-hCG levels are taken 48 hours apart.
  - In viable pregnancies the β-hCG level will more than double in 48 hours.
    ○ one-third of ectopic pregnancies also demonstrate this pattern.
  - Slower rising or declining levels of β-hCG are suggestive of an ectopic pregnancy.

Gynaecology

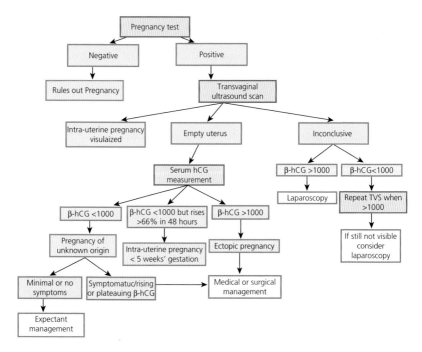

Fig. 16.1 Algorithm for the investigation of suspected ectopic pregnancy. hCG, human chorionic gonadotrophin; TVS, transvaginal ultrasound scan.

– All viable pregnancies should be visualized if the β-hCG level is above 1500 iu:
  ○ if the β-hCG level is greater than 1500 iu and the pregnancy is not visible, medical management can be considered;
  ○ if the β-hCG level is below 1500 iu, the ultrasound scan should be repeated when it rises above this level.

MICRO-facts

If the woman is haemodynamically unstable, a laparotomy is performed.

● **Treatment**:
  ● Initial management:
    – Most women are haemodynamically stable but all women are at risk of rapid deterioration; therefore, in symptomatic women the following steps are essential:

- ○ keep nil by mouth;
- ○ large-bore intravenous access;
- ○ full blood count (FBC) and cross-match;
- ○ consider anti-D prophylaxis (see Chapter 3, Medical problems in pregnancy).
  - – If haemodynamically unstable, begin fluid resuscitation and call for senior support.
- ● Expectant management:
  - – Some ectopic pregnancies terminate spontaneously.
  - – In women with no acute symptoms whose β-hCG < 1000 iu and continues to fall, conservative management may be an option.
  - – These women should be followed up twice weekly until β-hCG < 20 iu.
- ● Medical:
  - – Methotrexate (a folate antagonist):
    - ○ this is suitable for ectopic pregnancies that are unruptured, < 3 cm in diameter, and with a β-hCG level < 3000 iu;
    - ○ β-hCG levels are subsequently monitored to ensure that all the trophoblastic tissue has been destroyed. In some circumstances a second dose or surgery may be required;
    - ○ the dose depends on the patient's body surface area and is $50 \, mg/m^2$.
- ● Surgical:
  - – Laparoscopic salpingotomy:
    - ○ this is the gold standard;
    - ○ the ectopic is removed from the tube;
    - ○ there is a higher risk of residual trophoblast with this procedure than with laparotomy;
    - ○ this is the first-line surgical management for women who wish to have future pregnancies.
- ● Laparotomy:
  - – Performed if the patient is haemodynamically unstable.
  - – The ectopic and affected fallopian tube is also removed (salpingectomy).

MICRO-facts

Laparoscopic surgery is preferable to a laparotomy because recovery is faster and subsequent fertility rates are better.

Gynaecology

- **Prognosis**:
  - only 70% of women will subsequently have an intra-uterine pregnancy following an ectopic;
  - 10% of women will have another ectopic pregnancy.

> **MICRO-reference**
> Royal college of Obstetricians and Gynaecologists. The management of tubal pregnancy. Green Top Guideline no. 21. London, UK: RCOG, 2004. Available at http://www.rcog.org.uk/files/rcog-corp/GTG21_230611.pdf

16.2 MISCARRIAGE

- **Definition**:
  - spontaneous pregnancy loss before fetal viability, i.e. 24 completed weeks' gestation.
- **Epidemiology**:
  - occurs in 15–20% of clinical pregnancies.
- **Aetiology**:
  - The majority are due to a one-off chromosomal abnormality of the embryo.
  - The rarer causes are discussed in Recurrent miscarriage (see later).
- **Clinical features**:
  - 75% of miscarriages occur before 12 weeks' gestation.
  - There are four clinical presentations of miscarriage:
    - **Threatened**:
      - there is light vaginal bleeding but the fetus is still viable;
      - fetal death will occur in approximately 50% of cases;
      - the cervical os is closed.
    - **Inevitable**:
      - presents with heavy bleeding and pain;
      - the cervical os is open;
      - fetal death is inevitable.
    - **Missed**:
      - fetal death has occurred but the products of conception have not been expelled. It is often subclinical, and discovered incidentally on routine ultrasound scan.
    - **Recurrent**:
      - this is explored in Recurrent miscarriage (see later).
  - Miscarriage may also be described as:
    - **Complete**: all the products of conception have been expelled from the uterus. This usually occurs for gestations <8 weeks.
    - **Incomplete**: some products of conception are retained.

Table 16.1 Clinical features of miscarriage.

	DEFINITION	CLINICAL FEATURES				UTERINE SIZE	FETAL HEART BEAT ON TVS?
			PAIN	BLEEDING	CERVICAL OS		
Threatened	Bleeding from the genital tract before 24 weeks' gestation		Usually painless or mild pelvic cramping	Scanty, brownish discharge or bright red blood	Closed	As expected for dates	Yes
Missed	A gestational sac containing a non-viable fetus is detected on USS before 20 weeks' gestation.		None	None or minimal	Closed	Small for dates	No
Inevitable	Miscarriage is taking place. Although a fetal heart beat may be seen, the cervical os is open so fetal death is inevitable		Severe pelvic cramping	Heavy, with clots and tissue	Open	As expected for dates	Yes or no

Gynaecology

Table 16.1 (*Continued*)

	DEFINITION	CLINICAL FEATURES			UTERINE SIZE	FETAL HEART BEAT ON TVS?
		PAIN	BLEEDING	CERVICAL OS		
Complete	Miscarriage has occurred. All products of conception have been expelled from the uterus and bleeding has stopped	No	Minimal	Closed	Small/as expected for dates	No; uterus is empty
Incomplete	Miscarriage has occurred, but some products of conception are retained	Yes or no	Heavy	Open	Small/as expected for dates	No. Retained products are seen

TVS, transvaginal ultrasound scan; USS, ultrasound scan. Based on data from: http://www.gpnotebook.co.uk/simplepage.cfm?
ID = 523567157&linkID = 31448&cook = yes.

- **Investigations**:
  - TVS: to assess the location and viability of the pregnancy.
  - Serum/urine β-hCG:
    - if the pregnancy is viable, serum β-hCG will increase by 60–100% over 48 hours.
  - FBC and rhesus status.
  - Triple swabs if the woman is pyrexial.

MICRO-facts

If bleeding is heavy, resuscitation may be required.

- **Management**:

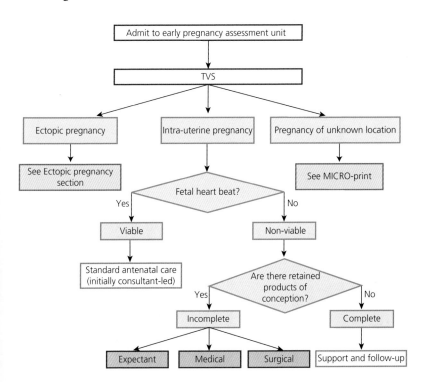

Fig. 16.2 Algorithm for the management of suspected miscarriage. TVS, transvaginal ultrasound scan.

Table 16.2 Comparison of management options for miscarriage.

	PROCEDURE	ADVANTAGES	DISADVANTAGES/COMPLICATIONS
Expectant	Patient returns home to pass the products of conception. She must stay where she can access 24 hour care quickly if symptoms worsen or if signs of infection occur	Hospitalization and risks of surgery avoided	• Vaginal bleeding may be heavy and take longer to resolve • Pain • Risk of incomplete miscarriage and need for surgery • Lower efficacy rate than medical/surgical management
Medical	Prostaglandins ± anti-progesterone (mifepristone) are given to induce abortion	Risks of surgery avoided	• More pain and bleeding than with surgery Pain and bleeding may persist for up to 3 weeks • Risk of incomplete miscarriage and need for surgery
Surgical	Evacuation of retained products of conception: suction curettage of the uterus under local or general anaesthetic	Rapid resolution of symptoms	• Perforation • Cervical tear • Intra-abdominal trauma • Intra-uterine adhesions • Asherman's syndrome • Haemorrhage and infection • Risks and complications of general anaesthetic

MICRO-print
In 10% of suspected miscarriages human chorionic gonadotrophin (β-hCG) is positive but the pregnancy cannot be located on transvaginal ultrasound scan (TVS). This is known as a **pregnancy of unknown location**. Cautious management with TVS, serial serum β-hCG and progesterone levels is essential as the pregnancy may be ectopic and rupture.

MICRO-facts
Anti-D should be given to rhesus-negative women with bleeding after 12 weeks' gestation and after surgical management of miscarriage.

MICRO-print
Asherman's syndrome is characterized by the presence of intra-uterine adhesions. It is an uncommon complication of uterine curettage. It may cause amenorrhoea and fertility problems.

MICRO-reference
Royal College of Obstetricians and Gynaecologists. The management of early pregnancy loss. Green Top Guideline no. 25. London, UK: RCOG, 2006. Available at http://www.rcog.org.uk/files/rcog-corp/uploaded-files/GT25ManagementofEarlyPregnancyLoss2006.pdf

16.3 RECURRENT MISCARRIAGE

- **Definition**:
    - three or more consecutive miscarriages.
- **Epidemiology**:
    - affects 1% of women.
- **Aetiology**:
    - Unknown in 50% of cases.
    - Parental genetic abnormalities, e.g. a balanced structural chromosomal anomaly.
    - Maternal anti-phospholipid syndrome.
    - Structural uterine anomaly.
    - Bacterial vaginosis (BV) may be implicated in late miscarriage (>16 weeks).

- Cervical incompetence:
  - there may be a history of cervical surgery or late termination of pregnancy;
  - causes recurrent late miscarriage.
- **Risk factors**:
  - higher maternal age;
  - previous miscarriage.
- **Investigations**:
  - parental karyotyping;
  - cytogenetic analysis of miscarried fetal tissue;
  - maternal anti-phospholipid antibody screen;
  - maternal pelvic USS;
  - in high-risk women (with a history of late miscarriage or spontaneous pre-term labour) BV screening and treatment should take place in early pregnancy.
- **Management**:
  - psychological counselling;
  - genetic counselling if chromosomal anomalies are detected;
  - anti-phospholipid syndrome: prescribe low-dose aspirin and low-dose heparin during future pregnancies;
  - manage underlying uterine anomalies accordingly;
  - cervical incompetence: consider cervical cerclage.
- **Prognosis**:
  - 75% of women will have a successful future pregnancy with psychological counselling alone.

MICRO-reference

Royal College of Obstetricians and Gynaecologists. The investigation and treatment of couples with recurrent miscarriage. Evidence-Based Clinical Guideline no. 17. London, UK: RCOG, 2003. Available at http://www.rcog.org.uk/womens-health/clinical-guidance/investigation-and-treatment-couples-recurrent-miscarriage-green-top-

---

16.4 GESTATIONAL TROPHOBLASTIC DISEASE

- **Definition**:
  - a group of disorders encompassing benign disease (complete and partial moles) and malignant conditions (invasive moles and choriocarcinoma).

Table 16.3 Comparison of complete and partial moles.

CHARACTERISTIC	COMPLETE MOLE	PARTIAL MOLE
Origin	Diploid (entirely paternal)	Triploid (maternal and paternal)
Fertilization	Usually one sperm fertilizing an empty ovum	Two sperm fertilizing one ovum
Presence of fetal tissue	No	Yes

- **Benign disease:**
  - **Hydatidiform mole (molar pregnancy):**
    - excessive proliferation of placental trophoblastic tissue that remains localized and non-invasive;
    - hydatidiform moles may be complete or partial (see Table 16.3).

> **MICRO-print**
> Trophoblastic tissue is the part of the blastocyst that invades the endometrium during implantation.

- **Malignant disease:**
  - **Invasive mole:**
    - excessive proliferation of placental trophoblastic tissue which is invasive but remains confined to the uterus.
  - **Choriocarcinoma:**
    - excessive proliferation of placental trophoblastic tissue, resulting in metastasis.
- **Epidemiology:**
  - very rare;
  - more common in Asian women and at extremes of reproductive age.
- **Clinical features of gestational trophoblastic disease (GTD):**
  - irregular vaginal bleeding;
  - hyperemesis (excessive vomiting);
  - uterine enlargement (greater than expected for gestational age);
  - early failed pregnancy;
  - hyperthyroidism (rarer);
  - early pre-eclampsia (rarer).
- **Investigations:**
  - Ultrasound:
    - typically shows 'snow-storm' appearance with complete moles (see Fig. 16.3).

Gynaecology

- Serum β-hCG:
  - may be greatly raised.
- The definitive diagnosis is histological.

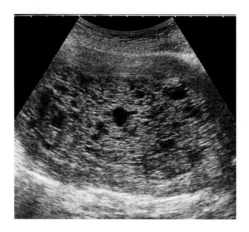

Fig. 16.3 Ultrasound scan showing 'snow-storm' appearance of molar pregnancy. Reproduced with permission from Monga A. *Gynaecology by Ten Teachers, 18th edn.* London: Hodder Arnold, 2011.

- **Management**:
  - suction curettage to remove trophoblastic tissue;
  - medical evacuation is used if the size of fetal parts in a partial molar pregnancy prevents suction curettage;
  - confirmation of histological diagnosis guides further management.
- **Complications**:
  - Recurrence of GTD in subsequent pregnancies (about 1:80).
  - GTD may become persistent. Persistent GTD is called gestational trophoblastic neoplasia (GTN):
    - diagnosis of GTN is made by a persistently elevated β-hCG level;
    - GTN may be malignant, e.g. choriocarcinoma. Symptoms include persistent vaginal bleeding or evidence of metastatic disease, e.g. dyspnoea.
- **Follow-up**:
  - All women with GTD are registered at a specialist centre that can guide management and screen for GTN by measuring serial serum or urinary β-hCG levels. If β-hCG levels normalize, the chance of developing GTN is low.

Gynaecology

- Women with GTN may be treated with single-agent or multi-agent chemotherapy:
  - prior to chemotherapy, women are assessed using the FIGO scoring system;
  - low-risk women only require single-agent therapy, e.g. intramuscular methotrexate.
- All women on the register should be screened after any future pregnancy.
- **Prognosis**:
  - in the UK, the cure rate is 98–100%;
  - chemotherapy is needed in only 5–8%.

MICRO-print

The specialist centres for gestational trophoblastic disease in the UK are in London, Sheffield and Dundee.

MICRO-reference

Royal College of Obstetricians and Gynaecologists. The management of gestational trophoblastic disease. Green Top Guideline no. 38. London, UK: RCOG, 2010. Available at http://www.rcog.org.uk/files/rcog-corp/GT38ManagementGestational0210.pdf

Gynaecology

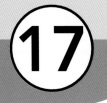

17 Termination of pregnancy (induced abortion)

17.1 INTRODUCTION

- **Definition**:
  - removal of the products of conception in order to terminate a pregnancy.
- **Epidemiology**:
  - one-third of British women will have had an induced abortion by the time they are 45 years old.
- **The Abortion Act**:
  - Under the 1967 Abortion Act (amended by the Human Fertilisation and Embryology Act 1990), induced abortion is legal in England, Scotland and Wales up to the **24th week** of pregnancy.
  - **Two doctors** must agree that the pregnancy satisfies one of five criteria (see Statutory grounds for induced abortion in Great Britain). The majority of procedures are carried out under part C.

MICRO-print
Fetal viability

- The legal definition of fetal viability is any fetus ≥24 weeks' gestation.
- Babies born earlier than this have a low chance of survival.
- From 24 weeks' gestation, a paediatrician must assess the baby at birth and resuscitate them if necessary.
- Before 24 weeks there is no legal requirement to carry out resuscitation.
- However, babies born at earlier gestations (<24 weeks) have survived in the past.
- The Nuffield Council on Bioethics (http://www.nuffieldbioethics.org/) provides guidance on these issues.

MICRO-facts

Statutory grounds for induced abortion in Great Britain

A. The continuance of the pregnancy would involve risk to the life of the pregnant woman greater than if the pregnancy were terminated.

B. The termination is necessary to prevent grave permanent injury to the physical or mental health of the pregnant woman.

C. The pregnancy has not exceeded its 24th week and the continuance of the pregnancy would involve risk, greater than if the pregnancy were terminated, of injury to the physical or mental health of the pregnant woman.

D. The pregnancy has not exceeded its 24th week and the continuance of the pregnancy would involve risk, greater than if the pregnancy were terminated, of injury to the physical or mental health of the existing child(ren) of the family of the pregnant woman.

E. There is a substantial risk that if the child were born it would suffer from such physical or mental abnormalities as to be seriously handicapped.

Data based on the Human Fertilisation and Embryology Act 1990. Available at http://www.legislation.gov.uk/ukpga/1990/37/section/37 © Crown Copyright.

MICRO-reference

The Abortion Act 1967. Available at http://www.legislation.gov.uk/ukpga/1967/87/section/1

Human Fertilisation and Embryology Act 1990. Available at http://www.legislation.gov.uk/ukpga/1990/37/section/37

17.2 PRE-ABORTION CARE

- Blood tests:
  - haemoglobin;
  - ABO and rhesus status.

MICRO-print

In at-risk groups, women should be tested for haemoglobinopathies, human immunodeficiency virus, and hepatitis B and C.

Gynaecology

- **Preventing infectious complications**:
  - antibiotic prophylaxis (e.g. metronidazole + doxycycline);
  - triple swabs.
- **Contraception counselling**:
  - discuss post-abortion contraception, so that it can be started immediately.

MICRO-facts

Termination of pregnancy is a potential sensitizing event. Rhesus-negative women should be given anti-D within 72 hours of the procedure.

17.3 METHODS OF ABORTION

There are three main methods of abortion:
1. medical abortion;
2. vacuum aspiration;
3. surgical abortion by dilatation and evacuation (D&E).

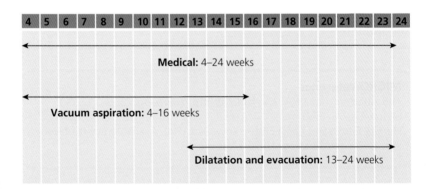

Fig. 17.1 Method of abortion by gestation. Adapted from Royal College of Obstetricians and Gynaecologists Clinical Guideline no. 7.

MICRO-reference

Royal College of Obstetricians and Gynaecologists. The care of women requesting induced abortion clinical. Clinical Guideline no. 7. London, UK: RCOG, 2011. Available at http://www.rcog.org.uk/files/rcog-corp/Abortion%20guideline_web_1.pdf

Gynaecology

- **Medical abortion**:
    - This is the most effective method of induced abortion below 9 weeks' gestation.
    - The oral anti-progesterone mifepristone is given to disimplant the fetus.
    - 36–48 hours later, a prostaglandin, e.g. misoprostol, is given orally or vaginally.
        - multiple doses may be needed for pregnancies of higher gestation.
    - The woman passes the pregnancy later that day.
    - Beyond 22 weeks' gestation, feticide (using KCl) is used to prevent live birth.
- **Vacuum aspiration**:
    - A suction curette is used to remove the products of conception under local or general anaesthetic.
    - Since there is no sharp instrumentation of the uterus, potential damage is minimal.
- **Surgical abortion by D&E**:
    - D&E is performed under a general anaesthetic after preparing the cervix with prostaglandin.
    - This method has the greatest risk of complications.

17.4 COMPLICATIONS OF ABORTION

- **Common complications**:
    - Genital tract infection.
    - Cervical trauma:
        - moderate risk in surgical abortions.
- **Less common complications**:
    - Haemorrhage:
        - low risk.
    - Incomplete abortion:
        - some products of conception may be retained following abortion. If these are not passed spontaneously surgical evacuation is required. Very rarely, the pregnancy will continue.
    - Uterine perforation:
        - low risk in surgical abortions.
    - Uterine rupture:
        - very low risk in mid-trimester medical abortions.
- There is **no evidence** of a causal association with:
    - psychiatric illness;
    - self-harm;
    - subsequent ectopic pregnancy, placenta praevia or infertility.

Gynaecology

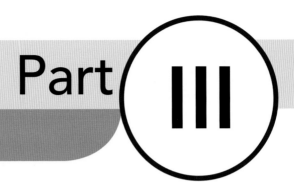

Part III

Women's health

18 Contraception

18.1 HORMONAL CONTRACEPTION

COMBINED ORAL CONTRACEPTIVE PILL

- Contains oestrogen and progesterone.
- **Mechanism of action**:
    - suppression of the pituitary gland preventing ovulation;
    - thickening of the cervical mucus;
    - thinning of the endometrium.
- **Failure rates**: 0.3 per 100 women years (if taken properly!).

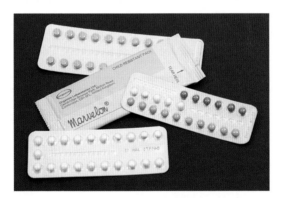

Fig. 18.1 Combined oral contraceptive pill.

MICRO-facts

Efficacy of contraception is measured using the Pearl index. This is a statistical estimation of the number of unintended pregnancies in 100 women years of exposure. If the Pearl index of a contraceptive is 1 then, 1 woman out of 100 using it for a year will be pregnant by the end of the year.

- **Directions for use**:
  - a single tablet is taken every day for 3 weeks;
  - with most types of pill there is a 7 day break in the fourth week; however, some types have a fourth week of placebo pills;
  - during the fourth week a withdrawal bleed usually occurs.
- **Contraindications**:
  - smokers ≥ 35 years;
  - history of venous thrombosis;
  - migraine with aura or migraine without aura and age ≥ 35 years;
  - active breast or endometrial cancer.

Table 18.1 Advantages and disadvantages of the combined oral contraceptive pill.

ADVANTAGES	DISADVANTAGES
Reversible and reliable	Increased risk of myocardial infarction and venous thrombosis (rare)
12 hour window in which to remember to take the pill	Drug interactions reduce efficacy (e.g. antibiotics, carbamazepine)
Reduces menorrhagia and dysmenorrhoea	Vomiting/diarrhoea reduces effectiveness
Reduces risk of pelvic inflammatory disease, endometrial and ovarian cancers	Can cause side-effects, e.g. nausea, headaches, breast tenderness
May help with acne	Medical history may not make everyone suitable (smokers, clots, migraine)

PROGESTERONE-ONLY PILL

- **Mechanism of action**:
  - makes cervical mucus hostile to sperm;
  - thinning of the endometrium;
  - may stop ovulation (15–40% women).
- **Failure rates**: 3 per 100 women years (higher than with the COCP).
- **Directions for use**:
  - must be taken at the same time every day (± 3 hours) without a break.

MICRO-facts

Cerazette® is a newer type of progesterone-only pill, which, like the combined oral contraceptive pill, has a 12 hour window of action.

Table 18.2 Advantages and disadvantages of the progesterone-only pill.

ADVANTAGES	DISADVANTAGES
Can be used in women who are not suitable for COCP (migraine, hypertension, obese)	Small window can spell failure if not meticulous with timing (3 hours; 12 hours for Cerazette®)
Can use while breast-feeding	Can cause side-effects (e.g. nausea, headaches, weight gain)
Reduces menorrhagia and dysmenorrhoea	Erratic bleeding in some women
Reversible and effective	Avoid if taking liver enzyme-inducing medication
Not affected by broad-spectrum antibiotics	

COCP, combined oral contraceptive pill.

MICRO-print

Some patients may want advice on what to do if they miss some of their pills. For up-to-date guidelines, please see the Family Planning Association website (http://www.fpa.org.uk).

CONTRACEPTIVE INJECTION (Depo-Provera® and Noristerat®)

- Long-acting reversible contraceptive.
- **Mechanism of action**:
    - progesterones are slowly released, bypassing the portal circulation;
    - cervical mucus becomes hostile to sperm and, unlike the POP, ovulation is usually also prevented.
- **Failure rate**: <0.4 in 100 women over 2 years.
- **Directions for use**:
    - Depo-Provera® is administered every 12 weeks by intramuscular injection;
    - Noristerat® is administered every 8 weeks.

Table 18.3 Advantages and disadvantages of the contraceptive injection.

ADVANTAGES	DISADVANTAGES
High efficacy rate	Irregular and prolonged bleeding in the first few weeks
Not user dependent	Side-effects (headaches and skin problems) will last as long as the injection lasts
Can use while breast-feeding	May be a delay in return to normal fertility (for up to 2 years!)
55% of women amenorrhoeic after 1 year	Decrease in bone density (regained on stopping)
	Increased appetite leads to weight gain in those who respond by 'snacking'

SUBDERMAL CONTRACEPTIVE IMPLANT (NEXPLANON®)

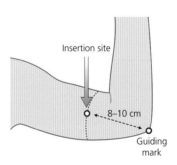

Fig. 18.2 Insertion position of Nexplanon®.

- A long-acting progesterone-only implant.
- It is radio-opaque and can be found by radiography.
- **Mode of action**:
  - similar to that of the POP and Depo-Provera®.
- **Failure rate**: <0.1 in 100 women over 3 years.
- **Directions for use**:
  - a 40 mm long and 2 mm wide plastic rod is inserted subdermally in the upper arm with a local anaesthetic (see Fig. 18.2);
  - it is important that the patient checks the rod herself after insertion.
- It lasts for 3 years.

Table 18.4 Advantages and disadvantages of Nexplanon®.

ADVANTAGES	DISADVANTAGES
Reversible and effective	Irregular bleeding in one-third of women
Long lasting and not user dependent	Progestogenic side-effects
Fertility returns rapidly	Requires a minor operation for insertion and removal
No decrease in bone density	
Causes amenorrhoea in one-third of women	
Can be used while breast-feeding	

> **MICRO-reference**
> National Institute For Health and Clinical Excellence. Long-acting reversible contraception: the effective and appropriate use of long-acting reversible contraception. London, UK: NICE, 2005. Available at http://www.nice.org.uk/nicemedia/live/10974/29912/29912.pdf

CONTRACEPTIVE PATCH

- Contains oestrogen and progesterone.
- **Mode of action**:
  - prevents ovulation;
  - increases cervical mucus thickness.
- **Failure rate**: 1 per 100 women years.
- **Directions for use**:
  - a small patch is applied to the skin;
  - a new patch is used each week for three weeks out of four.

Table 18.5 Advantages and disadvantages of the contraceptive patch.

ADVANTAGES	DISADVANTAGES
Reversible and reliable	May be visible
Easy to use	Increased risk of venous thrombosis
Not affected by diarrhoea or vomiting	Breakthrough bleeding and spotting are common in the first few months
Reduces dysmenorrhoea and menorrhagia	May cause side-effects including headache, nausea and breast tenderness in first few months

Women's health

EMERGENCY CONTRACEPTIVE PILL

- The 'morning-after pill' consists of 1.5 mg of levonorgestrel (a progestogen).
- **Mode of action**:
  - affects sperm function;
  - reduces endometrial receptivity;
  - may prevent follicular rupture if given prior to ovulation.
- **Directions for use**:
  - a single dose of levonorgestrel must be taken within 72 hours of unprotected intercourse and preferably within 24 hours.
- **Success rate**:
  - this depends on the time after unprotected intercourse that it is taken;
  - if taken within 24 hours it has a 95% success rate;
  - by 72 hours the success rate has fallen to 58%.

18.2 BARRIER METHODS

MECHANISM OF ACTION

- Prevent sperm from entering the cervix and reaching the ovum.
- Usually used in combination with a spermicide.

MALE CONDOM

- A sheath made of latex or polyurethane.
- **Directions for use**:
  - the sheath is unrolled onto an erect penis while pinching the end in order to expel air, which prevents splitting on ejaculation;
  - it should be put on before penetration and worn for the duration.
- **Failure rate**: 2 per 100 women years but can be as high as 15 if not used correctly.

FEMALE CONDOM

- **Directions for use**:
  - this is put inside the vagina;
  - it is held in place by a ring at each end.
- **Failure rate**: 5 per 100 women years but can be much higher owing to user failure.
- They are rarely used.

Table 18.6 Advantages and disadvantages of the male condom.

ADVANTAGES	DISADVANTAGES
Protects against STIs (but not those affecting the perineum)	Can interrupt sex
Easily available and free in many places	Can split or slip off
Only needs to be used during sexual intercourse	Latex or spermicide sensitivity
No side-effects unless latex allergy	

Table 18.7 Advantages and disadvantages of the female condom.

ADVANTAGES	DISADVANTAGES
Protects against STIs (but not those affecting the perineum)	Can interrupt sex
Effective	
Only need to use them during intercourse (can be inserted up to 8 hours beforehand)	May be difficult to insert
No lubricating gel required	Penis may pass alongside, rather than into it
	Can be noisy (!)
	Expensive to buy

IUCD, intra-uterine coil device; STI, sexually transmitted infection.

DIAPHRAGMS AND CAPS

- Not widely used in the UK.
- **Directions for use**:
  - **diaphragm**: covers the cervix and is held in place by the spring, between the pubic bone and sacrum;
  - **cap**: fits over the cervix;
  - inserted <2 hours before intercourse and must remain in place for >6 hours after intercourse;
  - must be used with spermicidal pessaries;
  - require professional fitting initially.
- **Failure rate**: 4–8 per 100 women years.

Table 18.8 Advantages and disadvantages of the diaphragm/cap.

ADVANTAGES	DISADVANTAGES
Provides some protection against some STIs	Requires forward planning
Less interruption of sex than condoms	Requires fitting
No loss of sensation	Increased risk of UTI
	Not as effective as other methods

STI, sexually transmitted infection; UTI, urinary tract infection.

18.3 INTRA-UTERINE DEVICE AND SYSTEM

OVERVIEW

- These are plastic devices that are inserted into the uterine cavity.
- A plastic thread protrudes through the cervix, which enables them to be removed.
- Intra-uterine coil device (IUCD or 'coil') contains copper.
- Intra-uterine system (IUS or Mirena®) contains progesterone.

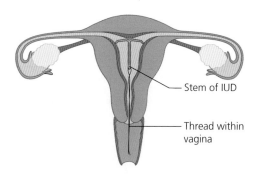

Stem of IUD

Thread within vagina

Fig. 18.3 Intra-uterine coil device (IUCD) in the uterine cavity.

INTRA-UTERINE COIL DEVICES

- **Mechanism of action**:
  - the copper is spermicidal and also prevents migration of the sperm;
  - implantation is also prevented.
- **Directions for use**:
  - the coil is inserted and removed by a medical professional;
  - it can be inserted at any time during the menstrual cycle provided it is reasonably certain the woman is not pregnant;

- women are encouraged to check for the presence of the strings after each period (owing to the risk of expulsion);
- follow-up after the first period and at 3 months as most expulsions occur in this time frame;
- changed every 5–10 years.
- **Failure rate**: <2 in 100 women over 5 years.
- **Use as an emergency contraceptive**:
  - prevents 99% of pregnancies (more effective than hormonal contraception);
  - it can be inserted within 5 days of unprotected intercourse (or within 5 days of likely ovulation if intercourse was more than 5 days previously);
  - prevents implantation and may have a toxic effect, preventing fertilization.

INTRA-UTERINE SYSTEM (Mirena®)

- **Mechanism of action**:
  - progesterone is released slowly and locally from the rod;
  - cervical mucus is thickened;
  - endometrium is thinned;
  - ovulation may be suppressed in some women;
  - implantation less likely to occur.
- **Directions for use**:
  - similar to the IUCD (see above);
  - must be changed every 5 years.
- **Failure rate**: <1 in 100 women over 5 years.

MICRO-facts

When counselling women on long-acting reversible contraception the following should be considered:

- contraceptive efficacy;
- duration of use;
- risks and possible side-effects;
- non-contraceptive benefits;
- the procedure for initiation and removal/discontinuation;
- when to seek help while using the method.

Women's health

Table 18.9 Advantages and disadvantages of the intra-uterine coil device (IUCD)/ intra-uterine system (IUS).

ADVANTAGES	DISADVANTAGES
Long-lasting and reversible	Expulsion
Effective	IUCD: menstruation can be longer and more painful
No interactions with other medications	IUS: irregular bleeding
No delay in return to fertility	Women with asymptomatic STIs are at increased risk of PID
Does not interrupt sex	Increased risk of ectopic if pregnancy occurs
IUS reduces menorrhagia	Perforation on insertion (rare)

PID, pelvic inflammatory disease; STI, sexually transmitted infection. (Source: James Trussell, Professor of Economics and Public Affairs at the University of Princeton)

> **MICRO-reference**
> National Institute for Health and Clinical Excellence. Long-acting reversible contraception: the effective and appropriate use of long-acting reversible contraception. London, UK: NICE, 2005. Available at http:// www.nice.org.uk/nicemedia/live/10974/29912/29912.pdf

18.4 NON-REVERSIBLE METHODS

FEMALE STERILIZATION

- **Procedure**:
    - occlusion of the fallopian tubes, thereby preventing union of the sperm and ovum;
    - usually performed laparoscopically using Filshie clips, with the patient under general anaesthesia;
    - a pregnancy test should be performed pre-operatively.
- **Failure rate**:
    - 3 in 1000;
    - if performed during termination of pregnancy or caesarean section, the failure rate is 7–20 in 1000; women should be told this prior to sterilization under these conditions.
- **Important points to consider before sterilization**:
    - Alternative methods of contraception: sterilization failure rates are no better than those for the new IUCDs.

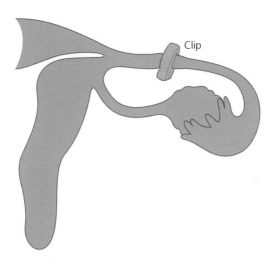

Fig. 18.4 **Female sterilization.**

- Reversal is not always successful and is not available on the National Health Service.
- Vasectomy is a safer procedure than female sterilization.
- Increased risk of ectopic pregnancy if pregnancy does occur.
- Risks of surgery:
  - visceral damage;
  - inadequate tubal access;
  - in the event of either of the above a laparotomy may be required, which carries further risks.

MALE STERILIZATION

- **Procedure**:
  - the vas deferens is ligated and a small section removed – this prevents sperm from being released;
  - can be performed as an outpatient under a local anaesthetic;
  - it is much simpler to perform than female sterilization.
- **Failure rate**:
  - 1 in 2000 (much more effective than female sterilization).
- **Important points to consider prior to sterilization**:
  - Complications of procedure:
    - haematoma;
    - infection;
    - failure;
    - chronic testicular pain.
  - Reversal is possible but not guaranteed to be successful.

- It may take 6 months for the ejaculate to become free of sperm; therefore, other methods of contraception must be used until there have been two ejaculates negative for sperm (taken 4 weeks apart).

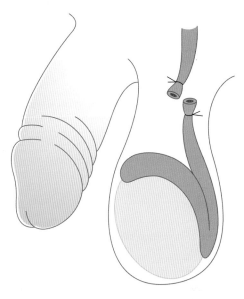

Fig. 18.5 Male sterilization.

18.5 SUMMARY OF CONTRACEPTION EFFICACY

Table 18.10 Percentage of women with unintended pregnancy in first year of contraceptive use.

CONTRACEPTIVE	PERFECT USE (%)	TYPICAL USE (%)
Spermicide	18	29
Diaphragm + spermicide	6	16
Male condom	2	15
Pill	0.3	8
Depo-Provera®	0.3	3
Nexplanon®	0.05	0.05
Mirena® IUS	0.2	0.2
Copper IUCD	0.6	0.8

19 Genital tract infections

19.1 SEXUAL HISTORY

PRESENTING COMPLAINT

Symptoms may include:

- warts;
- rash;
- itching;
- discharge;
- inter-menstrual bleeding;
- abdominal/pelvic pain;
- dyspareunia (superficial/deep);
- bleeding during/after sex.

    Also, consider whether:

- the symptoms are acute/chronic;
- the partner is symptomatic.

PAST HISTORY OF SEXUALLY TRANSMITTED INFECTIONS

- Which infection?
- When?
- Was it successfully treated?
- Was the partner is successfully treated?

LAST SEXUAL INTERCOURSE

- When did the patient last have sex?
- Was it with a regular sexual partner or a one-off?
- **Establish**:
    - gender;
    - type of sexual activity;
    - condom use;
    - nationality of sexual partner.

PREVIOUS SEXUAL PARTNERS

- When did the patient last have sex with someone other than that partner?
- Establish details for each partner, as above.
- Repeat for all sexual partners in the past 3–6 months.

CONTRACEPTION

- Is the patient currently using contraception?
  - Which form?
  - Discuss factors that may have affected the contraceptive's effectiveness, e.g. vomiting with the oral contraceptive pill.
- How long has the patient been using this type of contraception?

DRUG HISTORY

- Especially antibiotics in the last month.

RISK FACTORS FOR HUMAN IMMUNODEFICIENCY VIRUS

- History of intravenous drug use or of sex with an intravenous drug user.
- Having sex abroad (except with a travel partner).
- Sex with a man who has ever had a male sexual partner.
- Blood transfusion.

> **MICRO-print**
> When asking about unprotected sex, 'When did you last have sex without a condom?' is more likely to elicit an honest answer than 'Do you use condoms?'

19.2 NON-SEXUALLY TRANSMITTED INFECTIONS

CANDIDIASIS (THRUSH)

- **Epidemiology**:
  - vulvovaginal candidiasis affects more than 75% of women at some point in their lifetime.
- **Pathophysiology**:
  - infection with *Candida albicans* is the most common cause;
  - *Candida* may overgrow, causing an infection; this can be triggered by a disturbance to the normal flora;
  - it is not necessarily sexually transmitted.

- **Risk factors**:
  - pregnancy;
  - diabetes;
  - antibiotics.
- **Symptoms**:
  - 'cottage cheese' discharge;
  - itching;
  - superficial dyspareunia and dysuria may occur.
- **Signs**:
  - vulval irritation may cause the vulva to look red and inflamed.
- **Diagnosis**: microscopy and culture.
- **Treatment**:
  - topical imidazoles;
  - oral fluconazole.

BACTERIAL VAGINOSIS

- **Epidemiology**:
  - prevalence is $\sim 12\%$.
- **Pathophysiology**:
  - the lactobacilli that normally colonize the vagina are overgrown by a mixed flora of predominantly anaerobes.
- **Symptoms**:
  - grey–white discharge;
  - fishy odour;
  - vaginal epithelium is not inflamed.
- **Diagnosis**:
  - increased vaginal pH;
  - typical discharge;
  - positive 'whiff' test (a whiff of ammonia is detected when an alkali is added to a slide);
  - presence of 'clue cells' on microscopy.
- **Treatment**: clindamycin cream or metronidazole.
- **Complications**:
  - increased risk of pre-term labour;
  - may cause secondary infection in pelvic inflammatory disease (PID).

FOREIGN BODIES

- Foreign bodies may cause an offensive vaginal discharge.
- In children and those with learning difficulties it is important to consider sexual abuse.

Women's health

> **MICRO-print**
> **Toxic shock syndrome** can be caused by retention of foreign bodies (e.g. tampons) in the vagina.
> - It is a rare condition but can be fatal (10% mortality).
> - Symptoms may include: fever, diarrhoea, vomiting and an erythematous rash.

19.3 VAGINAL DISCHARGE ALGORITHM

See Fig. 19.1.

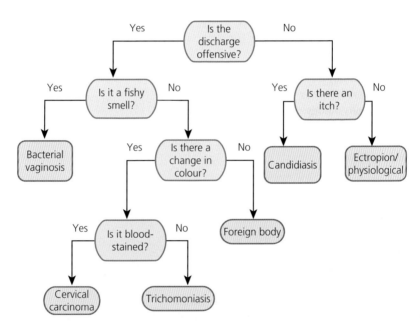

Fig. 19.1 Summary of the causes of vaginal discharge.

19.4 SEXUALLY TRANSMITTED INFECTIONS

TRICHOMONAS

- **Epidemiology**:
  - common worldwide;
  - less common than Chlamydia and gonorrhoea.

- **Pathophysiology**:
  - *Trichomonas vaginalis* is a flagellate protozoan that is transmitted sexually.
- **Symptoms**:
  - offensive grey–green discharge;
  - vulval irritation;
  - superficial dyspareunia;
  - can be asymptomatic.
- **Diagnosis**:
  - wet film microscopy.
- **Treatment:** metronidazole.

CHLAMYDIA

- **Epidemiology**:
  - approximately 5–10% of women <24 years are affected.
- **Pathophysiology**:
  - sexual transmission of the obligate intra-cellular organism *Chlamydia trachomatis* through penetrative sex.
- **Symptoms and signs**:
  - usually asymptomatic;
  - vaginal discharge;
  - post-coital bleeding or inter-menstrual bleeding;
  - urethritis;
  - lower abdominal or pelvic pain.
- **Diagnosis**:
  - Nucleic acid amplification tests:
    - Samples can be obtained in the following ways:
      - ○ endocervical swab;
      - ○ urine: first-catch specimen.
- **Treatment**:
  - azithromycin: single dose;
  - doxycycline: 14 day course.
- **Complications**:
  - PID: this can cause tubal damage leading to subfertility and/or chronic pelvic pain;
  - reactive arthritis, including Reiter's syndrome: a triad of urethritis, conjunctivitis and arthritis;
  - problems in pregnancy, including early miscarriage and premature birth.

Women's health

MICRO-facts

Untreated Chlamydia infection has serious complications, including infertility. Since infection is often asymptomatic, opportunistic screening identifies most cases. The National Chlamydia Screening Programme (http://www.chlamydiascreening.nhs.uk/ps/index.html) targets sexually active people <25 years in healthcare settings and in the community. The test is a urine sample or lower vaginal swab, which women do themselves. Screening should be annual or after a change in sexual partner.

GONORRHOEA

- **Epidemiology**:
    - most common in young adults (15–25 years of age);
    - has decreased in prevalence by 11% from 2007 to 2009;
    - co-infection with Chlamydia is identified in 35% of heterosexual men and 41% of women.
- **Pathophysiology**:
    - *Neisseria gonorrhoeae* (a Gram-negative diplococcus) is the causative organism.
- **Symptoms and signs**:
    - Usually asymptomatic in women.
    - Urethritis is common in men.
    - Other features include:
        - vaginal discharge;
        - bartholinitis;
        - cervicitis.
- **Diagnosis**: microscopy and culture of an endocervical swab.
- **Treatment**:
    - ceftriaxone: a single dose is the treatment of choice;
    - penicillin and ciprofloxacin can also be used;
    - most centres treat people diagnosed with gonorrhoea for Chlamydia also, regardless of swabs.
- **Complications**:
    - PID;
    - problems in pregnancy including spontaneous abortion and conjunctivitis in the newborn.

MICRO-print

Triple swabs are taken to identify lower genital tract infections. They comprise:

- One **high vaginal swab** of the vaginal fornix: to identify bacterial vaginosis, *Candida* and *Trichomonas*.
- Two **endocervical swabs**: the swab is inserted inside the cervical os and rotated against the endocervix.
    - A standard endocervical swab is tested for gonorrhoea.
    - A specific swab is used to test for Chlamydia.

MICRO-reference

http://www.chlamydiascreening.nhs.uk/ps/index.html
http://www.cks.nhs.uk/chlamydia_uncomplicated_genital/management/
scenario_chlamydia_uncomplicated_genital/partner_notification
http://www.cks.nhs.uk/gonorrhoea/management/scenario_gonorrhoea/
partner_notification
http://www.cetl.org.uk/learning/skills_sheets/Gynae-triple-swabs.pdf

MICRO-print

Partner notification is carried out for confirmed cases of Chlamydia and gonorrhoea to prevent reinfection and avoid complications. Sexual contacts are notified by the patient themselves or by a healthcare professional. Notified partners receive sexually transmitted infection screening and empirical treatment for gonorrhoea and Chlamydia.

MICRO-reference

http://www.cks.nhs.uk/gonorrhoea/
http://www.cks.nhs.uk/chlamydia_uncomplicated_genital

GENITAL WARTS (CONDYLOMATA ACCUMINATA)

- **Epidemiology**: very common.
- **Pathophysiology**:
    - Caused by the human papillomavirus (HPV):
        - types 6 and 11.
    - It is usually transmitted by sexual contact but can also be spread by autoinoculation from hand to genitals.

Women's health

- **Appearance**:
    - usually painless lumps which vary in appearance from tiny and flat to papilliform (see Fig. 19.2).
- **Distribution**:
    - tend to affect the vulva and introitus but may also affect the cervix.
- **Treatment**:
    - topical podophyllin (contraindicated in pregnancy);
    - imiquimod cream (external warts);
    - cryotherapy or electrocautery if resistant.
- **Complications**:
    - may also be exposed to HPV types 16 and 18, which are associated with the development of cervical intra-epithelial neoplasia;
    - high recurrence rate.

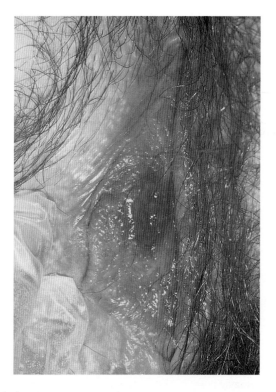

Fig. 19.2 Genital warts.

GENITAL HERPES

- **Epidemiology**:
  - The rate of diagnosis is higher among women than among men for primary genital herpes: affects 43:100 000 women and 29:100 000 men.
- **Pathophysiology**:
  - Caused by the herpes simplex virus (HSV)
  - There are two types:
    - HSV 1: can affect oral and genital areas;
    - HSV 2: affects the genitals.
  - Primary infection is usually the most severe; however, some people are initially asymptomatic and only later develop symptoms.
  - The virus subsequently lies dormant in the dorsal root ganglia.
  - Reactivations occur in 75%: these are usually less severe.
  - The virus can be passed on to partners even when asymptomatic and is therefore often passed on unknowingly.

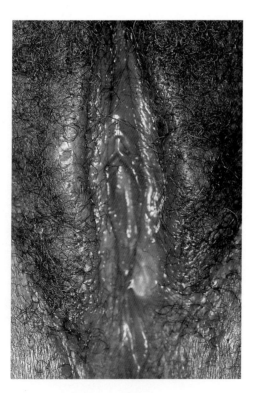

Fig. 19.3 **Primary herpes.**

- **Signs and symptoms**:
  - multiple, painful ulcers around the introitus (see Fig. 19.3);
  - local lymphadenopathy;
  - dysuria;
  - systemic symptoms: fever and myalgia.
- **Diagnosis**:
  - viral swab of the lesion.
- **Treatment**:
  - aciclovir: used in severe infections and will reduce the duration of symptoms if started early in a reactivation.
- **Complications**:
  - aseptic meningitis with/without encephalitis;
  - acute urinary retention;
  - neonatal herpes; for more information, see Chapter 3, Medical problems in pregnancy.

SYPHILIS

- **Epidemiology**: the number of new cases has increased dramatically.
- **Pathophysiology**:
  - Infection with the bacterium *Treponema pallidum* (see Fig. 19.4).
  - There are several stages:

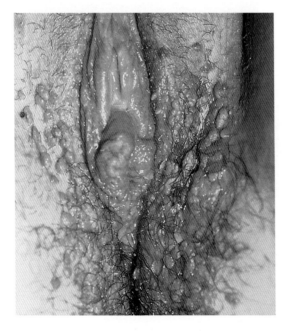

Fig. 19.4 **Syphilis**.

- Primary syphilis: formation of a solitary painless ulcer (chancre).
- Secondary syphilis: develops 1–6 months later if primary syphilis is not treated. Influenza-like symptoms develop and there may be a rash.
- Latent syphilis: secondary syphilis has resolved by this stage and is now asymptomatic.
- Tertiary syphilis: very rare and develops many years later. Many organs can be affected resulting in: aortic regurgitation, dementia, tabes dorsalis, gummata in the skin and bone.

- **Diagnosis**: Venereal Disease Research Laboratory testing.
- **Treatment**: penicillin.

PELVIC INFLAMMATORY DISEASE

- **Definition**:
  - Infection of the female upper genital tract, i.e. one or more of the following:
    - endometritis;
    - salpingitis;
    - parametritis;
    - oophoritis;
    - tubo-ovarian abscess;
    - pelvic peritonitis.
- **Epidemiology**:
  - most common in young, sexually active women; diagnosed in 1.7% of GP attendances by women aged 16–46 years.
- **Pathophysiology**:
  - Ascending infection from the lower genital tract.
  - Almost all cases of PID are due to Chlamydia or gonorrhoea:
    - spread to the pelvis is usually spontaneous, but may be a complication of uterine instrumentation;
    - complications of childbirth and miscarriage may also be implicated but tend to introduce non-sexually transmitted bacteria.
  - Vaginal commensals may also be implicated.
- **Symptoms**:
  - may be asymptomatic (particularly chlamydial);
  - bilateral lower abdominal/pelvic pain;
  - deep dyspareunia;
  - abnormal vaginal bleeding;
  - abnormal vaginal or cervical discharge.
- **Signs**:
  - Fever ($>38°C$).
  - Lower abdominal tenderness, usually bilateral:
    - may have some rebound tenderness.
  - On bimanual vaginal examination:

Women's health

- uterine tenderness;
- adnexal tenderness with/without adnexal mass;
- cervical excitation.

- **Diagnosis**:
  - based on clinical signs and symptoms;
  - do a pregnancy test to rule out ectopic pregnancy;
  - take triple swabs; confirming gonorrhoea or Chlamydia supports the diagnosis **but** negative swabs do not rule out PID;
  - consider a laparoscopy if symptoms do not improve with treatment after 48 hours.

- **Management**:
  - Treat empirically with broad-spectrum antibiotic therapy to cover *C. trachomatis*, *N. gonorrhoeae*, aerobic and anaerobic vaginal commensals, e.g. ceftriaxone + doxycycline + metronidazole.
    - antibiotic regime may depend on local geographical sensitivities.
  - Give appropriate analgesia.
  - Admit if febrile, systemically unwell or in a surgical emergency.

- **Complications**:
  - tubal factor infertility;
  - ectopic pregnancy;
  - chronic pelvic pain.

MICRO-print

In 10–20% of women with pelvic inflammatory disease, infection may spread intra-abdominally to cause peri-hepatitis, known as **Fitz–Hugh–Curtis syndrome**. Adhesions form between the liver and the peritoneum, presenting as right upper quadrant pain.

MICRO-case

A 24-year-old woman presented to her GP with a 4 day history of lower abdominal pain, mucopurulent discharge and fever. The discomfort had gradually worsened and she was taking regular paracetamol with some benefit. Her last menstrual period had been 2 weeks previously and she had not had any inter-menstrual bleeding.

She was single and had been taking the combined oral contraceptive pill for 2 years. She had had multiple sexual partners during this time and occasionally used condoms. She had not had any investigations for sexually transmitted infections.

continued...

continued...

On examination, she had a heart rate of 82 b.p.m., blood pressure of 110/76 mmHg and a temperature of 37.4°C. On palpation of her abdomen, it was soft with some generalized tenderness on light palpation in the lower quadrants. On bimanual examination there was cervical and adnexal tenderness. On speculum examination the cervix appeared slightly inflamed and some mucopurulent discharge was noted in the vagina. High vaginal, endocervical and urethral swabs were taken. A pregnancy test was negative.

The clinical features are suggestive of acute pelvic inflammatory disease. As there were no signs of generalized sepsis and the patient thought that the pain was sufficiently controlled with paracetamol and non-steroidal anti-inflammatory drugs, the GP decided to commence outpatient antibiotic therapy, consisting of oral ofloxacin and metronidazole.

The GP arranged follow-up for 72 hours' time in order to ensure that there was demonstrable clinical improvement. The patient was given advice regarding the use of barrier contraception and contact tracing of present and previous partners.

Key points:

- A detailed sexual history should be taken.
- Chlamydial and gonococcal infections are commonly implicated.
- Positive swabs support the diagnosis. Negative ones do not exclude it.
- It is important to consider other causes such as ectopic pregnancy and appendicitis.
- Admission is required in cases of generalized sepsis and if there is a poor response to oral treatment.
- Advice on the use of barrier contraception, until the infection is completely cured, should be given.
- Current and previous partners should be contacted and screened.

MICRO-reference

Ross J. UK national guideline for the management of pelvic inflammatory disease. Available at http://www.bashh.org/documents/118/118.pdf

HUMAN IMMUNODEFICIENCY VIRUS

A thorough exploration of human immunodeficiency virus (HIV) and acquired immunodeficiency syndrome (AIDS) is beyond the scope of this book. A brief overview of the gynaecological manifestations of HIV and AIDS is given.

- Genital conditions associated with HIV infection:
  - Chronic HPV infection:

Women's health

- – Genital warts.
- HIV-positive women are at greater risk of cervical neoplasia:
  - – annual cervical screening is recommended;
  - – invasive cervical cancer is an AIDS-defining illness in a HIV-positive individual.
- HIV-positive women are at greater risk of vulval intra-epithelial neoplasia.
- Herpes simplex infection:
  - – recurrent or large ulcers may indicate HIV infection;
  - – an ulcer that persists for more than 1 month is AIDS defining.
- PID.
- Vaginal candidiasis.
- Molluscum contagiosum.
- HIV/AIDS and contraception:
  - condoms and lubrication are advised to prevent HIV transmission, but an additional method of contraception is required to avoid pregnancy;
  - anti-retroviral therapy may make hormonal contraception less effective;
  - the intra-uterine coil device may increase the risk of PID for HIV-positive women.
- HIV testing is now part of routine antenatal screening.

MICRO-facts

For more information on a patient's medical eligibility for contraception, refer to: World Health Organization. Medical eligibility criteria for contraceptive use, 4th edn. Geneva, Switzerland: WHO, 2009. Available at http://www.who.int/reproductivehealth/publications/family_planning/9789241563888/en/index.html

MICRO-reference

British Association for Sexual Health and HIV, British HIV Association and British Infection Society. Guidelines for HIV testing. London, UK: BASHH, BHVA and BIS, 2008. Available at http://www.bashh.org/documents/1742/1742.pdf

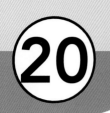

Diseases of the breast and their assessment and treatment
Sally Hallam

20.1 IMPORTANT FEATURES IN A BREAST HISTORY

PATIENT'S AGE

- Benign and malignant breast diseases are more likely in certain age groups.

MENOPAUSAL STATUS

- Levels of circulating oestrogen affect the breast tissue.

PARITY

- Parity, early pregnancy and breast-feeding reduce a woman's relative risk of developing breast cancer.

BREAST-FEEDING HISTORY

- Breast-feeding women are more prone to periductal mastitis and galactoceles.

RELATIONSHIP OF SYMPTOMS TO MENSTRUAL CYCLE

- Cyclical breast pain and nodularity are usually symptoms of benign aetiology.

BREAST LUMP

- Is there a discrete lump or is the breast generally lumpy (nodularity)?
- Is the lump fixed or mobile?
- Is the lump painful? This suggests a benign aetiology.
- Duration of the lump?
- Associated features:
    - skin tethering?
    - nipple retraction?

BREAST PAIN (MASTALGIA)

- Duration.
- Severity.
- Is the pain related to the menstrual cycle?
- Is the pain related to physical activity?
  - muscular pain in the pectoral or serratus anterior may mimic breast pain.
- Is the pain localized to the sternal edge?
  - costochondritis may present as breast pain.

NIPPLE DISCHARGE

- Bilateral or unilateral?
- Is the discharge from a single duct or multiple ducts?
  - Bilateral, multiduct discharge is very common and is usually due to duct ectasia.
  - Does the discharge appear spontaneously or only when the nipple is expressed?
  - Is the discharge bloodstained?
    - this requires further investigation as it may indicate a papilloma, infection, pre-cancerous change or cancer.

NIPPLE RETRACTION

- Some women have long-standing nipple inversion (Fig. 20.1); however, recent onset may be a sign of cancer.

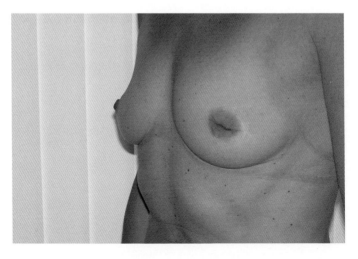

Fig. 20.1 Nipple retraction. Reproduced with permission from Abrahams PH, Craven JL, Lumley JSP. *Illustrated clinical anatomy*, 2nd edn. London: Hodder Arnold, 2010.

CHANGE IN SKIN CONTOUR

- Peau d'orange which may be indicative of inflammatory breast cancer.

FAMILY HISTORY

- Incidence of breast or ovarian cancer in first-degree relatives.

20.2 EXAMINATION OF THE BREAST AND LYMPH NODES

EXAMINATION

Examination of the breast should be handled with sensitivity, respect and privacy:

- A chaperone should always be present.
- A gown should be available to cover the woman/man once the examination is complete.
- Ask if the breasts are tender before commencing.

INSPECTION

With the patient sitting in the three positions shown in Fig. 20.2:

- Resting the hands at the sides relaxes the pectoral muscles (Fig. 20.2a).
- Ask the patient to place their hands firmly on their hips and push in (Fig. 20.2c):
    - this contracts the pectoral muscles, which may reveal tethering or distortion.
- Ask the patient to place their hands above and behind their head (Fig. 20.2b):
    - this stretches the pectoral muscle and skin over the breast.
- Inspect the breasts for:
    - asymmetry;
    - swelling;
    - change in skin contour;
    - nipple retraction.

PALPATION

- Positioning:
    - position the patient semi-recumbent at 45°;
    - the patient's head should be supported on a pillow;
    - ask women with larger breasts to place their hands behind their head; this stretches the breast tissue over the chest wall, making examination easier.

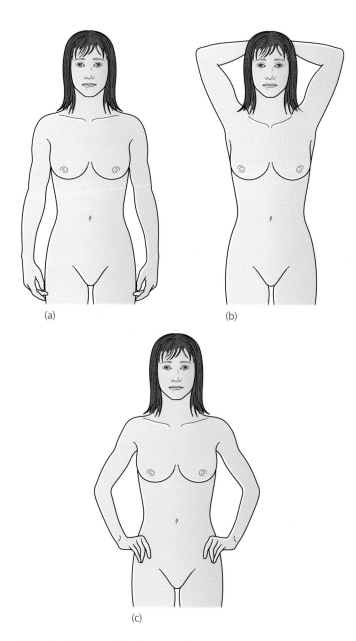

Fig. 20.2 (a–c) Patient position for breast inspection.

- Examine all areas of the breast, including upwards towards the clavicle and from the midline to the axilla.
- Initial palpation should be gentle to identify any tender areas.
- Use the flat of the fingertips to 'roll' the breast tissue against the chest wall. Do not pinch the tissue between finger and thumb.
- Be systematic and thorough. If you cannot find the lump, ask the patient to find it for you and examine again.
- If a mass is detected, determine its:
    - size;
    - position;
    - mobility;
    - consistency.
- Determine whether it is fixed to the chest wall or pectoral muscles (do this by gently moving the lump with the pectoral muscles relaxed or contracted).

LYMPH NODE EXAMINATION

- Support the full weight of the patient's right arm with your left hand and forearm to relax the muscles in the axilla (see Fig. 20.3a).
- Place the flat of your other hand in the axilla and compare the axillary contents against the chest wall, feeling for any palpable masses.
- To examine the left axilla, support the patient's arm with your right hand and forearm and repeat the process.
- Palpate the patient's supraclavicular nodes for any palpable masses (see Fig. 20.3b).
    - This is an infrequent site of metastasis.

20.3 BENIGN BREAST DISEASES

BREAST NODULARITY

- **Definition**:
    - benign breast change (previously known as fibroadenosis or fibrocystic change);
    - cyclical, nodular, often tender breasts.
- **Clinical features**:
    - bilateral cyclical pain and nodularity in a pre-menopausal woman.
- **Management**:
    - Mild:
        - reassurance and simple analgesia.
    - Severe (interferes with daily activities):
        - refer to breast clinic for evaluation;
        - endocrine therapies such as danazol or bromocriptine may be advised in the short term.

Women's health

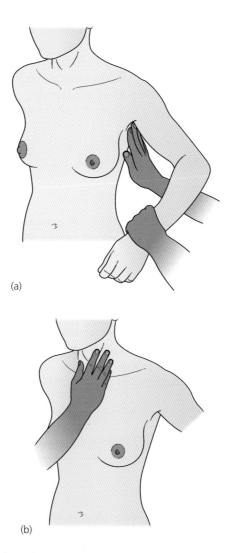

(a)

(b)

Fig. 20.3 Position for axillary and supraclavicular lymph node examination. (a) Axillary; (b) supraclavicular.

FIBROADENOMA (BREAST MOUSE)

- **Definition**:
  - Fibroadenomas are benign breast tumours composed of hyperplastic fibrous and glandular tissue; they account for 13% of all breast lumps.
- **Epidemiology**:
  - Fibroadenomas are the most common mass in women of childbearing age. Prevalence declines with age.

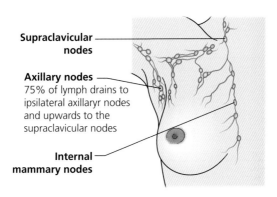

Supraclavicular nodes

Axillary nodes
75% of lymph drains to ipsilateral axillaryr nodes and upwards to the supraclavicular nodes

Internal mammary nodes

Fig. 20.4 Location of lymph node metastasis in breast cancer.

- **Clinical features**:
  - Oestrogen responsive; increase in size during pregnancy; and may be associated with cyclical pain:
    - a painless mass;
    - firm;
    - mobile;
    - clearly defined border on palpation.
- **Investigations**:
  - diagnosis is confirmed by core needle biopsy.
- **Management**:
  - fibroadenomas of >3 cm should be surgically removed.

BREAST CYSTS

- **Definition**:
  - a fluid-filled distended breast lobule.
- **Epidemiology**:
  - common in the peri-menopausal period (40–55 years).
- **Clinical features**:
  - smooth discrete breast lump;
  - with/without pain.
- **Investigations**:
  - mammogram: 'halo' sign;
  - ultrasound: fluid-filled cyst;
  - aspiration: blood-stained aspirate should prompt further investigation such as cytology.

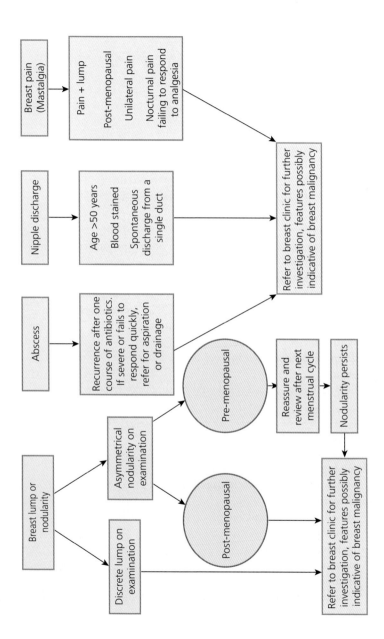

Fig. 20.5 Algorithm for the identification and referral of malignant breast disease.

- **Features suggesting an underlying malignancy**:
  - persistence of the lump after aspiration or repeated refilling;
  - a thick or irregular cyst wall;
  - blood-stained aspirate.

MASTITIS AND BREAST ABSCESS

- **Definition**:
  - common in breast-feeding women owing to blockage of milk ducts and bacteria entering the breast;
  - mastitis is inflammation of the breast;
  - it may lead to abscess formation (a collection of pus and necrotic tissue).
- **Aetiology**:
  - Lactation-associated abscesses are usually caused by *Staphylococcus aureus*. Those in non-lactating, usually older, women are generally linked to periductal mastitis and duct ectasia and are caused by a broader range of organisms.
- **Clinical features**:
  - flu-like symptoms;
  - breast pain;
  - swelling;
  - breast cellulitis;
  - breast lump.
- **Investigations**:
  - ultrasound;
  - aspiration.
- **Management**:
  - Surgical drainage.
  - Antibiotic therapy:
    - Lactational:
      - flucloxacillin (this is safe in lactating women);
      - erythromycin (for penicillin-allergic women).
    - Non-lactational:
      - amoxicillin/clavulanic acid.
  - Ultrasound-guided aspiration of the pus may hasten recovery and allow bacterial sensitivity to be determined.
  - Surgery: open incision and drainage under general anaesthesia is used in severe cases:
    - associated skin necrosis;
    - multiloculation;
    - persistence despite antibiotics.

Women's health

FAT NECROSIS

- **Definition**:
  - trauma to adipose tissue resulting in cell death and hydrolysis;
  - results in a solid mass.
- **Aetiology**:
  - may be associated with a history of trauma, e.g. seatbelt injury following a road traffic accident, although only 40% of women recall trauma to the breast.
- **Clinical features**:
  - mobile, firm mass;
  - clearly defined border;
  - breast pain or bruising.
- **Investigations**:
  - mammography or ultrasound;
  - biopsy or aspiration of liquid fat.
- **Management**:
  - often resolves spontaneously.

NIPPLE ECZEMA

- **Definition**:
  - eczema of the nipple.
- **Clinical features**:
  - commonly bilateral;
  - affects the areola but not the nipple (Fig. 20.6a).
- **Management**:
  - responds to moisturizers and steroid creams;
  - this should always be referred to the breast clinic as it can be a sign of Paget's disease of the nipple (see Breast cancer).

20.4 BREAST CANCER

EPIDEMIOLOGY

- Breast cancer is the most commonly diagnosed cancer in women in the UK.
- It affects 47 700 women in the UK per year and results in the death of 12 000.
- One in eight women in the UK will be diagnosed with breast cancer in their lifetime.
- The median age is 62, but any woman from the age of 18 may be affected.

AETIOLOGY

- Increasing age.
- Increased breast density.

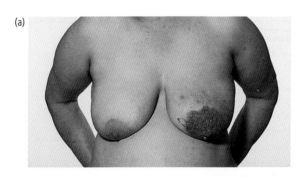

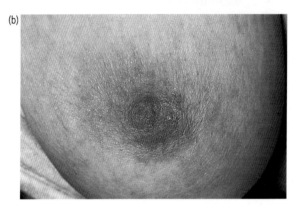

Fig. 20.6 (a) Nipple eczema and (b) Paget's disease of the nipple. Reproduced with permission from Black J, Thomas W, Burnand K, Browse N. *Browse's introduction to the symptoms and signs of surgical disease*, 4th edn. London: Hodder Arnold, 2005.

- Factors which increase cumulative lifetime oestrogen exposure:
  - early menarche;
  - low parity;
  - late first pregnancy;
  - late menopause;
  - hormone replacement therapy use;
  - use of the oral contraceptive pill;
  - obesity;
  - hereditary factors (see later).

CLINICAL FEATURES

- One-third of all breast cancers are asymptomatic and are diagnosed by routine mammographic screening.

Women's health

- Common presentations include:
  - A painless lump.
  - Distortion of the skin overlying the breast.
  - Nipple discharge or inversion.
  - Paget's disease of the nipple:
    - **Definition**:
      - a malignant condition which may be mistaken for nipple eczema;
      - Paget's disease is indicative of pre-cancerous cells tracking up the nipple ducts and infiltrating the dermis of the nipple.
    - **Clinical features**:
      - red scaly rash of the areola;
      - may be mistaken for nipple eczema: commonly unilateral, **always** affects the nipple rather than just the areola (Fig. 20.6b).
- Less commonly it may present with:
  - diffuse breast nodularity;
  - metastatic disease, e.g. a pathological fracture or jaundice.

SCREENING

- Breast cancer screening aims to detect breast tumours before they become clinically evident.
- Women are invited for mammographic screening every 3 years between the ages of 50 and 70.
- This age range is being extended to 47–73 in England between 2011 and 2013.
- Women over this age may attend voluntarily for as long as they wish to do so, but the benefits of screening reduce with increasing age so they are no longer routinely invited.

MICRO-facts

Mammography has high sensitivity for the investigation of breast disease in post-menopausal women owing to the high fat content and low density of their breasts. In pre-menopausal women the higher density of the breast tissue reduces mammography sensitivity. In women <35 years old, ultrasound or MRI can be used to image an area of concern.

FAMILIAL BREAST CANCER

- Breast cancer is sporadic in 70% of women, i.e. there is no underlying familial cause.
- For women at an increased familial breast cancer risk, screening with mammograms may commence at age 40.
- 5–10% of breast cancers are linked to one of several potent breast cancer genes, such as *BRCA1* and *BRCA2* (for these women screening MRI may commence at age 30).

MICRO-facts

It is estimated that screening reduces mortality from breast cancer by 25%. On average tumours detected by screening are smaller and less likely to require mastectomy than those presenting symptomatically. See http://www.cancerscreening.nhs.uk/breastscreen/

DIAGNOSIS

- Women with suspected breast cancer undergo triple assessment. This comprises:
    - clinical assessment and examination;
    - breast imaging (mammography and ultrasound);
    - biopsy (usually a core biopsy).
- Every suspected breast cancer case is reviewed by the breast multidisciplinary team to ensure that all three aspects of the triple assessment are concordant and to plan optimal treatment.
- **Breast imaging**:
    - A typical cancer found on a mammogram is shown in Fig. 20.7b.
    - Fig. 20.7a shows a normal mammogram:
        - there is fatty breast tissue, with scattered islands of fibroglandular tissue.
    - Fig. 20.7b is abnormal:
        - the arrow indicates a spiculated (irregularly shaped) mass with poorly defined margins; this is typical of cancer;
        - this is an invasive ductal carcinoma.
- **Biopsy**:
    - **Procedure**:
        - **Fine needle aspiration**: cells are aspirated using a fine needle and syringe; the architecture of the tumour is not preserved (it is not possible to identify where in the area of breast sampled the malignant cells have come from).
        - **Core needle biopsy**: a hollow needle is used to remove a solid sample of tissue with preserved architecture.

Women's health

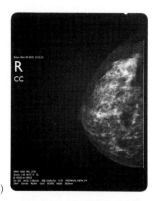

(a)

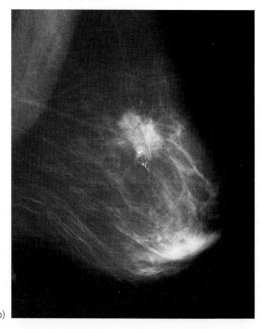

(b)

Fig. 20.7 A normal (a) and abnormal (b) mammogram. (a) © marcel - Fotolia.com. (b) Reproduced with permission from Neal and Hoskin. *Clinical Oncology*, 4th edn. London: Hodder Arnold, 2009.

- **Histological grading**:
  - Pathological samples are assessed by microscope and given a histological grade from 1 to 3 based on the degree of resemblance to the tissue of origin.
  - High tumour grade (poor resemblance to their tissue of origin) independently correlates with:
    - the development of distant metastasis;

– decreased breast cancer specific survival;
– shorter disease-free survival

- **Endocrine receptor status**:
  - Immunohistochemistry is used to assess the tumour sample for the expression of oestrogen receptor (ER) and human epidermal growth factor receptor 2 (HER2).
  - This information is combined with the patient's menopausal status to determine the appropriate endocrine adjuvant treatment.
- **TNM staging (see Table 20.1)**:
  - The tumour (T)–node (N)–metastasis (M) staging system for breast cancer combines the following investigations to assess the anatomical extent of the breast cancer:
    – tumour size;
    – lymph node status;
    – presence of distant metastasis.

MANAGEMENT OF PRIMARY OPERABLE BREAST CANCER

The stage of the tumour, its size in relation to the size of the breast, its receptor status (ER and HER2) and the fitness of the patient all determine management.

SURGERY

Breast-conserving surgery

- **Definition**:
  - removal of tumour and excision margin.
- **Indications**:
  - usually up to 20% of the breast can be removed;
  - if the volume of tissue removed is excessive, the breast may be distorted or shrink; breast reshaping may be required to minimize this.
- **Procedure**:
  - the tumour plus a 0.5–1 cm margin of normal breast tissue is removed from the breast;
  - after surgery a course of radiotherapy is given to the breast.
- **Prognosis**:
  - with this management there is a 10–12% risk of local recurrence at 20 years.

Mastectomy

- **Definition**:
  - removal of the whole of the breast.
- **Indications**:
  - large tumour relative to breast size, precluding breast conservation;
  - multifocal tumour;

Women's health

Table 20.1 TNM classification of breast tumours.

PRIMARY TUMOUR (T)	
TX	Primary tumour cannot be assessed
T0	No evidence of primary tumour
Tis	Carcinoma *in situ*: Ductal carcinoma *in situ* Lobular carcinoma *in situ* Paget's disease of the nipple with no invasive component
T1	Tumour ≤ 2 cm in greatest dimension
T2	Tumour ≥ 2 cm, < 5 cm
T3	Tumour is > 5 cm
T4	Tumour of any size with direct invasion into chest wall or skin
LYMPH NODE STATUS (N)	
NX	Unable to assess nearby lymph nodes
N0	No evidence of spread to nearby lymph nodes
N1	Metastasis in movable axillary lymph nodes
N2	Metastasis in fixed axillary lymph nodes Metastasis in fixed internal mammary nodes
N3	Metastasis in infraclavicular nodes $\pm$ axillary nodes/internal mammary nodes Metastasis in supraclavicular nodes $\pm$ axillary nodes/internal mammary nodes
METASTASIS (M)	
MX	Unable to assess for metastasis
M0	No evidence of metastasis
M1	Metastatic spread is evident

From Wittekind C, Greene FL, Hutter RVP, *et al.* TNM atlas: illustrated guide to the TNM/pTNM classification of malignant tumours. New York, NY: Springer, 2004, pp. 207–24.

- previous radiotherapy to the breast;
- patient choice.
- **Procedure**:
  - standard mastectomy incision: an elliptical area of skin is removed across the whole width of the breast (Fig. 20.8a);

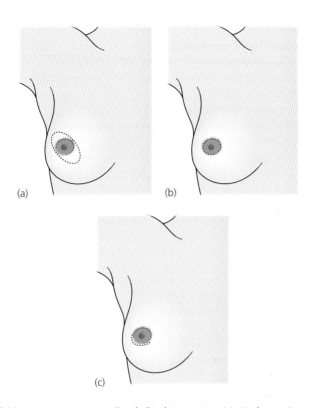

Fig. 20.8 Mastectomy types. (a) Total; (b) skin sparing; (c) nipple sparing.

- skin-sparing technique: the skin over the whole breast (Fig. 20.8b) and sometimes even the nipple (Fig. 20.8c) is preserved to permit good quality immediate reconstruction.
- Radiotherapy is recommended post-operatively for about 20% of women with tumours that are high grade and heavily node positive or large or inflammatory cancers (T3 or T4).

Reconstructive surgery

- **Indications:**
  - all women who require or request a mastectomy should be considered for reconstruction of the breast;
  - this can be delayed or immediate depending on the need for further treatment and the patient's wishes;
  - some women may be unfit for such complex surgery owing to co-morbid disease.

Women's health

- **Procedure**:
  - **Implant-based reconstruction**:
    - The insertion of a synthetic implant, usually made of silicone, either immediately or following a period of tissue expansion with a saline-filled implant.
  - **Autogenous reconstruction**:
    - Skin, muscle and fat from a donor site on the patient's back or abdomen is transferred to the breast.
    - The tissue is transferred as:
      - ○ a pedicled flap: the blood supply from the donor site is maintained;
      - ○ a free flap: the blood supply is disconnected and reconnected to a new blood vessel system near to the breast.

Axillary node surgery

- **Indications**:
  - all women undergoing breast-conserving surgery and mastectomy;
  - to identify axillary metastases.
- **Procedure for axillary biopsy**:
  - If the axillary lymph nodes appear normal, surgical sampling of a small number of nodes is undertaken. This may be done in one of two ways:
    - **Axillary node sampling**:
      - ○ the removal of four lymph nodes from the axilla, sampling those which are largest and nearest to the tumour;
      - ○ this technique has a false-negative rate of up to 5%.
    - **Sentinel lymph node biopsy**:
      - ○ the sentinel nodes are those that the tumour and the tissue surrounding it first drain into;
      - ○ blue-coloured and radioactive dyes are injected into the tissue surrounding the breast tumour;
      - ○ the dye drains first into the sentinel nodes (Fig. 20.9a);
      - ○ a probe is used to detect the absorbance of the dye by the sentinel nodes and these are removed;
      - ○ this allows more accurate detection of metastatic spread than by simply removing the nodes closest to the tumour.
- If metastatic lymph nodes are detected an axillary lymph node clearance is indicated.
- **Axillary node clearance**:
  - axillary node clearance involves the removal of all axillary lymph nodes and their surrounding adipose tissue;

(a)

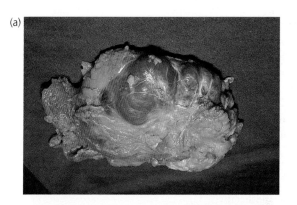

(b)

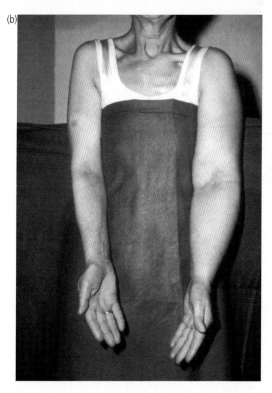

Fig. 20.9 (a) Sentinel lymph node biopsy. Reproduced with permission from Black J, Thomas W, Burnand K, Browse N. *Browse's introduction to the symptoms and signs of surgical disease*, 4th edn. London: Hodder Arnold, 2005. (b) Lymphoedema. Reproduced with permission from Abrahams PH, Craven JL, Lumley JSP. *Illustrated clinical anatomy*, 2nd edn. London: Hodder Arnold, 2010.

- clearance of the axillary nodes is associated with a 15% risk of lymphoedema of the arm;
- lymphoedema is a potentially permanent tissue swelling due to localized retention of lymphatic fluid (Fig. 20.9b).

ADJUVANT THERAPIES

- **Indication**:
  - Following on from surgery, many women are offered additional (or adjuvant) therapies to help reduce the risk of the cancer recurring either in the surgical scar or as systemic metastases.
  - There are four main types of adjuvant therapy for breast cancer:
    - radiotherapy;
    - chemotherapy;
    - endocrine therapy;
    - trastuzumab (Herceptin®).

Adjuvant Endocrine Therapy

- **Indication**:
  - All breast cancers are tested for their ER status to determine which adjuvant therapies should be used.
  - ER-positive tumours are treated with anti-oestrogen therapy.
  - **Pre-menopausal women** are treated with tamoxifen therapy for 5 years.
    - **Definition**:
      - tamoxifen blocks the effects of oestrogen by competitively inhibiting its action at the ER in breast tissue;
      - tamoxifen is a partial oestrogen agonist on bone and endometrial tissues.
    - **Side-effects**:
      - it is associated with an increased risk of endometrial cancer with long-term use and a decreased risk of osteoporosis.
  - In **post-menopausal women** the primary source of oestrogen production is conversion from androgens by aromatase in peripheral tissues. Treatment in this age group is with aromatase inhibitors (letrozole, anastrozole).
    - **Definition**:
      - aromatase inhibitors block the synthesis of oestrogen in post-menopausal women.

MICRO-facts

Tamoxifen therapy for 5 years is associated with a 9.2% reduction in breast cancer mortality and an 11.8% reduction in recurrence. See http://www.ctsu.ox.ac.uk/~ebctcg/

Adjuvant Trastuzumab

- **Indication**:
  - The epidermal growth factor receptor (EGFR2; HER2) is over-expressed in one-third of all breast cancers and is a poor prognostic factor.
  - Breast cells over-expressing the HER2 proteins show an uncontrolled rate of growth and behave very aggressively with a high rate of metastases.
  - Trastuzumab (Herceptin®) is a monoclonal antibody that binds to HER2 receptor proteins, reducing cell proliferation and tumour growth.
  - Trastuzumab is recommended for 12 months for women with HER2-positive breast cancers following chemotherapy treatment.
- **Prognosis**:
  - Trastuzumab treatment results in a 34% reduction in mortality compared with chemotherapy alone.

Adjuvant Chemotherapy

- **Indication**:
  - Chemotherapy is indicated in the adjuvant setting (after definitive surgical treatment) for those women with more aggressive cancers:
    - younger age;
    - high tumour grade;
    - nodal disease;
    - large primary cancer size;
    - ER-negative cancers and HER2-positive cancers.
- **Procedure**:
  - Chemotherapy regimes are complex but usually include the anthracycline doxorubicin (or epirubicin) and cyclophosphamide, with addition of a taxane for women with more aggressive cancers.
- **Side-effects**:
  - Mucocutaneous ulceration.
  - Nausea, vomiting.
  - Diarrhoea.

Women's health

- Hair loss.
- Fatigue.
- Infertility/premature menopause:
  - chemotherapy can result in premature ovarian failure, causing infertility and an increased risk of osteoporosis and cardiovascular disease;
  - regimens can be altered to preserve ovarian function in younger women;
  - patients may opt to freeze eggs, embryos or ovarian tissue to increase fertility options following treatment. (Of these options, only embryo storage is reliably effective and egg and ovarian tissue storage are still largely experimental.)
- More serious adverse events such as neutropenic sepsis and bleeding result from suppression of bone marrow function.

MICRO-reference

National Institute for Health and Clinical Excellence. Advanced breast cancer: diagnosis and treatment. NICE Clinical Guideline 81. London, UK: NICE, 2009.

Adjuvant Radiotherapy

- **Indications**:
  - following wide local excision; it reduces the risk of local recurrence from 35% to 10–12% in this situation;
  - patients undergoing mastectomy, with stage T3 or T4 tumours of high grade, four or more involved lymph nodes or involved resection margins.
- **Procedure**:
  - radiotherapy is given daily for a period of 3–5 weeks.
- **Side-effects**:
  - As radiotherapy is targeted to the breast, systemic side-effects are minimal.
  - **Acute side-effects** include:
    - fatigue;
    - local skin irritation;
    - oedema;
    - pain.
  - **Long term side-effects** include:
    - discoloration and fibrosis of the skin;
    - lymphoedema;
    - increased risk of cancer in the area treated 5–15 years later (1:1000 risk).

MICRO-reference

National Institute for Health and Clinical Excellence. Early and locally advanced breast cancer: diagnosis and treatment. NICE Clinical Guideline 80. London, UK: NICE, 2009.

National Institute for Health and Clinical Excellence. Advanced breast cancer: diagnosis and treatment. NICE Clinical Guideline 81. London, UK: NICE, 2009.

PSYCHOLOGICAL SUPPORT

- A diagnosis of breast cancer can be a traumatic and distressing experience for the patient and their family.
- A source of support is the breast care nurse. A breast care nurse sees every patient at the time of diagnosis, allowing a detailed discussion of his or her concerns.
- Breast care nurses provide education about breast cancer and its treatment as well as physical, practical, psychological and emotional support throughout the patient's treatment, referring for further help if needed.

20.5 LOCALLY ADVANCED BREAST CANCER

- **Definition**:
    - This term describes breast cancer that is surgically incurable at diagnosis. Features of locally advanced breast cancer include the following:
        - greater than 5 cm diameter;
        - fixed to the chest wall;
        - ulceration;
        - fixed axillary lymph nodes;
        - inflammatory breast cancer.
- **Management**:
    - Chemotherapy is used initially to downstage the tumour, allowing subsequent definitive surgical treatment with mastectomy.
    - This may be followed by adjuvant endocrine therapy or radiotherapy.

20.6 METASTATIC BREAST CANCER

- **Definition**:
    - Metastatic breast cancer is the systemic spread of tumour cells to distant organs from the breast and axillary lymph nodes.

Women's health

- **Prognosis**:
  - Palliative treatment can increase median survival by a number of years.
- **Management**:
  - Treatment is multimodal with anti-oestrogen adjuvant drugs for ER-positive cancers, trastuzumab (Herceptin®) for HER2-positive cancers and chemotherapy.
  - Breast cancer has the potential to metastasize to any part of the body; however, it commonly metastasizes to bone, followed by lung, liver and finally the brain.

MICRO-reference

National Institute for Health and Clinical Excellence. Early and locally advanced breast cancer: diagnosis and treatment. NICE Clinical Guideline 80. London, UK: NICE, 2009.

National Institute for Health and Clinical Excellence. Advanced breast cancer: diagnosis and treatment. NICE Clinical Guideline 81. London, UK: NICE, 2009.

BONE METASTASIS

- **Clinical features**:
  - Bone metastasis may be sclerotic or lytic:
    - pain;
    - pathological fracture;
    - spinal cord compression;
    - hypercalcaemia.
- **Management**:
  - Treatment is with endocrine therapy if the primary tumour was oestrogen sensitive.
  - Radiotherapy or surgery can be used to treat pathological fractures and bone pain.
  - Serum calcium levels must be regularly monitored as patients are at high risk of hypercalcaemia owing to the release of parathyroid hormone-related peptide by tumour cells or bone lysis.

LUNG METASTASIS

- **Clinical features**:
  - lung metastases present with pleural effusion or a lung mass.
- **Management**:
  - effusions can be drained if symptomatic and the pleural space obliterated to prevent recurrence (pleurodesis);
  - endocrine or chemotherapy can then be used to treat the metastasis.

LIVER METASTASIS

- **Clinical features**:
  - right upper quadrant pain or signs of liver failure.
- **Prognosis**:
  - liver metastases have a relatively poor prognosis with a median survival of 4 months.
- **Management**:
  - aggressive chemotherapy may increase survival to 1–2 years if the patient is medically fit for this.

BRAIN METASTASIS

- **Clinical features**:
  - headache or focal neurology.
- **Prognosis**:
  - brain metastases have the worse prognosis, with survival of only 1–2 months.
- **Management**:
  - treatment options include radiotherapy, high-dose steroids and surgery for solitary metastasis.

MICRO-reference

National Institute for Health and Clinical Excellence. Advanced breast cancer: diagnosis and treatment. NICE Clinical Guideline 81. London, UK: NICE, 2009.

20.7 PAGET'S DISEASE OF THE NIPPLE

- **Definition**:
  - a malignant condition that may be mistaken for nipple eczema.
  - paget's disease is indicative of pre-cancerous cells tracking up the nipple ducts and infiltrating the dermis of the nipple.
- **Clinical features**:
  - commonly unilateral, **always** affects the nipple rather than just the areola (Fig. 20.6b).

Women's health

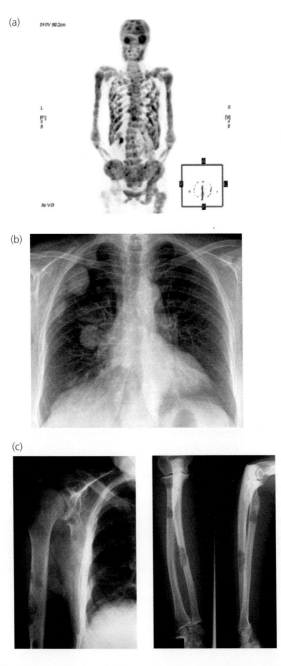

Fig. 20.10 Metastasis. (a) Isotope bone scan showing multiple 'hot spot' areas of high metabolic activity suggesting metastasis. (b) Lung radiograph showing typical cannonball metastasis. (c) Lytic metastasis in the radius (reproduced with permission from Neal and Hoskin, *Clinical Oncology* 4E. London: Hodder Arnold, 2009).

MICRO-case

A 59-year-old woman presented to her GP with a mass in the right breast; the mass had gradually increased in size over a 3 month period and was painless. The patient had no family history of breast cancer and no recent trauma to the chest.

On examination there was a 2 × 2.5 cm mass in the upper outer quadrant of the right breast with associated dimpling of the skin; no masses were palpable in the contralateral breast or either axilla.

The patient was sent to the one-stop breast clinic, where clinical examination mammography and fine needle aspiration were performed:

- Mammography: 2.2 × 2.8 cm spiculated mass in the right upper outer quadrant of the breast.
- Grade: 3 poorly differentiated.
- Endocrine receptor status: oestrogen receptor positive.

The patient was sent for a staging CT scan, which showed no distant metastasis; she then attended the breast clinic, where she discussed her options. The patient was concerned about the risk of tumour recurrence and opted for mastectomy with sentinel lymph node biopsy. Lymph node biopsy detected malignant lymph node spread and axillary clearance was performed on the right side.

TNM staging was determined to be T2, N2, M0. The patient went on to receive radiotherapy to the chest wall and adjuvant tamoxifen; 1 year post-operatively the patient decided to opt for a latissimus dorsi (LD) flap implant-assisted reconstruction.

Key points:

- Prompt referral to the breast clinic is important for accurate and timely diagnosis of breast cancer.
- Triple assessment and operative findings provide the basis for the TNM staging and grading systems.
- Treatment options must be a joint decision based on clinical indications and patient choice.
- All women undergoing mastectomy must be offered breast reconstruction surgery.

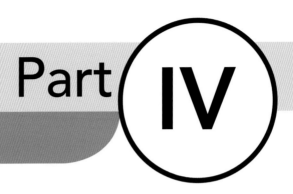

Part IV

Self-assessment

21 Obstetrics

Questions

EMQs

For each of the following questions, choose the most likely cause of obstetric haemorrhage. Each option may be used once, more than once or not at all.

Options:

<table>
<tr><td>1) Atonic uterus</td><td>6) Placental abruption</td></tr>
<tr><td>2) Cervical tear</td><td>7) Placenta praevia</td></tr>
<tr><td>3) Cervicitis</td><td>8) Retained products of conception</td></tr>
<tr><td>4) Endometritis</td><td>9) Uterine rupture</td></tr>
<tr><td>5) Perineal trauma</td><td>10) Vasa praevia</td></tr>
</table>

Question 1:

A 38-year-old woman (para 4) presents with vaginal bleeding 5 hours postpartum. She thinks that she has been losing blood slowly for an hour or so. She had an uncomplicated vaginal delivery. At 31 weeks she was diagnosed with polyhydramnios, for which no cause was identified. On examination the uterus is soft and at the level of the umbilicus.

Question 2:

A 29-year-old primiparous woman is 33 weeks pregnant with a single pregnancy. She presents with severe abdominal pain and dark vaginal bleeding. She has been bleeding for 5 hours and has lost approximately one sanitary towel's worth of blood. She was diagnosed with pre-eclampsia at 24 weeks. On examination she is tachycardic. Her abdomen is tender and the uterus is woody hard. Fetal heart sounds are diminished with decelerations.

Question 3:

A 40-year-old woman is 39 weeks pregnant with a single pregnancy. She presents with collapse and heavy, painless vaginal bleeding. She has a history of caesarean section for delivery of a twin pregnancy. On examination she is tachycardic and hypotensive. The fetus is in transverse lie.

For each of the following questions, choose the most likely infection. Each option may be used once, more than once or not at all.

Options:

1) Bacterial vaginosis
2) Cytomegalovirus
3) Gonorrhoea
4) Group B *Streptococcus*
5) Herpes simplex
6) Listeriosis
7) Parvovirus
8) Rubella
9) Toxoplasmosis
10) Varicella zoster

Question 4:

A protozoan infection that is commonly asymptomatic in the mother but can cause hydrocephalus or microcephaly if passed to the fetus. It can be transmitted in undercooked meat or cat faeces.

Question 5:

Causes a mild, flu-like illness in infected women. If transmitted to the fetus it may cause blindness, deafness and intra-uterine growth restriction.

Question 6:

Twenty-five per cent of women are carriers of this organism, which colonizes the vagina. In some women it is transmitted to the neonate during delivery, which can cause neonatal sepsis, meningitis and pneumonia.

SBAs

Question 7:

A 42-year-old multiparous woman is 38 weeks pregnant with a single pregnancy. She presents with vaginal bleeding and severe abdominal pain. On examination she is pale; the uterus is tender and hard. Ultrasound confirms that the placenta occupies the upper segment of the uterus. A cardiotocogram shows fetal tachycardia. What is the most appropriate mode of delivery in this case?
1) Admit and monitor with cardiotocography until the onset of labour
2) Elective caesarean section
3) Emergency caesarean section
4) Give steroids and induce labour
5) Induce labour

Question 8:

A 43-year-old nulliparous woman is pregnant after *in vitro* fertilization treatment. On the 20 week anomaly scan the placenta is found to occupy the lower segment of the uterus. A transvaginal scan confirms minor placenta praevia. She has not noticed any vaginal bleeding. Which of the following is the most appropriate management of this woman?

1) Deliver by caesarean section at 34 weeks
2) Deliver by elective caesarean section at 39 weeks
3) Normal vaginal delivery
4) Repeat transvaginal ultrasound at 32–36 weeks
5) Vaginal examination to confirm the position of the placenta

Question 9:

A 41-year-old nulliparous woman is seen in the antenatal clinic. She is 23 weeks pregnant and complains of headache and nausea. On examination her blood pressure is 172/110 mmHg and she has pedal oedema. A urine dipstick is positive for protein. This is confirmed by a 24 hour urine collection. A repeat blood pressure is recorded at 174/112 mmHg. Which of the following drugs is the most appropriate treatment of this woman's hypertension?

1) Atenolol
2) Labetalol
3) Losartan
4) Magnesium sulphate
5) Ramipril

Question 10:

A 32-year-old woman who is 39 weeks pregnant presents to the maternity unit with regular contractions every 3 minutes. She is para 1 with one previous normal vaginal delivery at term. On vaginal examination the membranes are intact. The cervix is fully effaced and 3 cm dilated. Three hours later her cervix is dilated to 7 cm. Delivery is expected in the next 2–3 hours. Entonox is not adequately controlling her pain. She has no known medical problems. What is the most appropriate form of analgesia?

1) Epidural
2) Labouring in water
3) Pethidine
4) Pudendal block
5) Spinal

Question 11:

A 28-year-old primiparous woman with a known coagulopathy presents to the maternity unit with regular contractions every 5 minutes. On examination the cervix is effaced and dilated 4 cm. Two hours later she is in a lot of pain despite

breathing and relaxation techniques and the use of Entonox. She would like further pain relief. What is the most appropriate form of analgesia?
1) Epidural
2) Pethidine
3) Pudendal block
4) Spinal
5) Transcutaneous electrical nerve stimulation

Question 12:

A 26-year-old woman (para 0) is clinically suspected of a breech presentation at 36 weeks. An extended breech is confirmed on ultrasound scan. What is the most appropriate management option?
1) Elective caesarean section
2) Emergency caesarean section
3) External cephalic version >37 weeks
4) Induction of labour
5) Planned vaginal delivery

Question 13:

Mrs X is a 42-year-old woman in her second pregnancy. Her first pregnancy was complicated with pre-eclampsia. She has a body mass index of 31. Serial ultrasound scans from 28 weeks show symmetrical growth restriction and this is confirmed on a fetal Doppler scan at 34 weeks. What is the most appropriate next step in management?
1) Delivery of the fetus
2) Fetal blood sampling
3) Intermittent auscultation
4) Monitoring with umbilical artery Doppler with/without daily cardiotocography
5) No intervention

Answers

EMQs

Answer 1:

1) **Atonic uterus:** this is the most common cause of postpartum haemorrhage. The uterus has failed to contract, so is large and soft on examination. It is more common in multiparous women and with polyhydramnios owing to uterine

overdistension. Active management of the third stage of labour (i.e. intramuscular oxytocin, controlled cord traction) reduces the risk of uterine atony. The uterus may require evacuation. See Atonic uterus in Chapter 7, Complications in labour.

Answer 2:

6) **Placental abruption:** this presents with painful vaginal bleeding. Although this woman has not visibly lost a large volume of blood, she is shocked. It is likely that she has concealed bleeding too. Pre-eclampsia and maternal smoking are key risk factors for abruption. The reduction in fetal blood supply has caused fetal distress. An urgent caesarean section is indicated. See Placental abruption in Chapter 7, Complications in labour.

Answer 3:

7) **Placenta praevia:** in contrast to placental abruption, vaginal bleeding from placenta praevia is **painless**. Blood loss can be profuse, causing hypovolaemic shock and maternal collapse. There is abnormal lie because the placenta is low lying. The fetal head cannot engage. Previous caesarean section and increasing maternal age are risk factors for placenta praevia. In practice, it is very rare for placenta praevia to present so late; commonly, it is identified by routine antenatal ultrasound scans. See Placenta praevia in Chapter 7, Complications in labour.

Answer 4:

9) **Toxoplasmosis:** this is the only protozoan and is found in cat faeces, soil or undercooked meat. See Toxoplasmosis in Chapter 3, Medical problems in pregnancy.

Answer 5:

2) **Cytomegalovirus** (CMV): this is often asymptomatic or causes mild, non-specific flu-like symptoms in the mother; blindness, deafness and growth restriction in the fetus. Rubella infection usually causes a febrile rash in the mother. Parvovirus may cause a flu-like illness; however, the most common presentation in the fetus is hydrops, which can be seen on an ultrasound scan. See Cytomegalovirus in Chapter 3, Medical problems in pregnancy.

Answer 6:

4) **Group B *Streptococcus*:** women are asymptomatic as it is a common vaginal commensal. Transmission can occur following rupture of the membranes and may cause neonatal sepsis. See Group B *Streptococcus* in Chapter 3, Medical problems in pregnancy.

SBAs

Answer 7:

3) **Emergency caesarean section:** placental abruption has occurred. First, the mother should be resuscitated if required. There is evidence of fetal distress; therefore, emergency caesarean section is required. Steroids are not needed after 34 weeks. See Placental abruption in Chapter 7, Complications in labour.

Answer 8:

4) **Repeat transvaginal ultrasound at 32–36 weeks:** in the majority of low-lying placentas discovered at 20 weeks the uterus stretches and the placenta moves upwards away from the cervix. A repeat ultrasound at 32–36 weeks will confirm this. If the placenta remains low lying, the mode and timing of delivery depends on the proximity of the placenta to the cervical os and whether any bleeding has occurred. See Placenta praevia in Chapter 7, Complications in labour.

Answer 9:

2) **Labetalol:** the patient has moderate pre-eclampsia ($>170/110\,mmHg$) requiring anti-hypertensive medication. Atenolol, ramipril and losartan are contraindicated in pregnancy. Magnesium sulphate is appropriate in this case but it is not an anti-hypertensive; rather, it increases cerebral perfusion to prevent eclampsia. Labetalol, nifedipine or hydralazine would be an appropriate choice. See Pre-eclampsia in Chapter 3, Medical problems in pregnancy.

Answer 10:

1) **Epidural:** this woman is in severe pain and should not be denied adequate pain relief. Since she has no known contraindications to epidural analgesia and is in the active first stage an epidural is the most appropriate option. Pethidine is not suitable given the proximity of delivery; it may cause neonatal respiratory distress. See Regional anaesthesia in Chapter 6, Labour.

Answer 11:

2) **Pethidine:** this woman has a coagulopathy; therefore, epidural anaesthesia is contraindicated. Pethidine can be used intravenously given the early stage of labour. See Opiates in Chapter 6, Labour.

Answer 12:

3) **External cephalic version >37 weeks** (ECV): as a breech presentation has been confirmed on ultrasound scan ECV is indicated. It is relatively safe and there are no contraindications in this case. ECV has been shown to reduce the

number of caesarean sections due to breech presentations. See Breech presentation in Chapter 7, Complications in labour.

Answer 13:

4) **Monitoring with umbilical artery Doppler with/without daily cardiotocography:** as the fetus is <37 weeks it is important to monitor for signs of placental dysfunction with Doppler and, if possible, hold off delivery until >37 weeks. However, if there are signs of fetal distress, delivery will be required earlier. Intermittent auscultation is of no benefit in this instance. See Doppler in Chapter 5, Fetal growth and surveillance.

Questions

EMQs

For each of the following questions, please pick the most appropriate management. Each option may be used once, more than once or not at all.

Options:

1) Abdominal ultrasound scan
2) Admit overnight and monitor
3) Discharge with appropriate analgesia
4) Expectant management
5) Laparoscopy
6) Laparotomy
7) Methotrexate
8) Monitor human chorionic gonadotrophin (β-hCG) levels
9) Repeat transvaginal ultrasound scan (TVS) in 1 week
10) TVS when β-hCG >1000

Question 1:

A 23-year-old woman who is pregnant (gestation approximately 7 weeks) presents with a 1 day history of colicky lower abdominal pain. You suspect an ectopic pregnancy and arrange a transvaginal ultrasound scan, which is inconclusive. Serum human chorionic gonadotrophin is 1800 iu.

Question 2:

A 34-year-old woman presents with a 2 day history of colicky lower abdominal pain and vaginal bleeding. She has not had a period for 6 weeks and a pregnancy test was positive. On examination her heart rate is 110 b.p.m. and her abdomen is tender on palpation. Blood pressure is 86/72 mmHg.

Question 3:

A 28-year-old woman is referred from her GP with a suspected ectopic pregnancy. She has a positive pregnancy test and a 1 day history of lower abdominal pain. She has had one previous ectopic pregnancy, which was treated with a salpingectomy. On examination her abdomen is soft and non-tender.

Transvaginal ultrasound scan reveals an empty uterus. Serum human chorionic gonadotrophin is 2051 iu. She would like to have more children in the future.

For each of the following questions, please pick the most appropriate first-line management. Each option may be used once, more than once or not at all.

Options:

1) Abdominal/pelvic ultrasound scan	6) MRI pelvis
2) Cervical smear	7) Pipelle biopsy
3) Colposcopy	8) Serum CA-125
4) CT abdomen	9) Transvaginal ultrasound
5) Hysteroscopy	10) Triple swabs

Question 4:

A 62-year-old woman presents to her GP with a 3 month history of post-menopausal bleeding.

Question 5:

A 28-year-old woman with a 1 month history of post-coital bleeding.

Question 6:

A 70-year-old woman with persistent abdominal pain, bloating and early satiety.

For each of the following questions, choose the most likely cause of menorrhagia. Each option may be used once, more than once or not at all.

Options:

1) Combined oral contraceptive pill	6) Hypothyroidism
2) Dysfunctional uterine bleeding	7) Intra-uterine coil device
3) Endometrial carcinoma	8) Ovarian tumour
4) Endometriosis	9) Pelvic inflammatory disease
5) Fibroids	10) Polycystic ovary syndrome

Question 7:

A 40-year-old Afro-Caribbean woman presents with a 12 month history of heavy periods. On examination there is a firm, irregular mass in the abdomen arising from the pelvis.

Question 8:

A 32-year-old woman presents with a 3 year history of heavy, painful periods. She complains of constant pain in her lower back and thighs, and deep dyspareunia. For the past 2 years she and her partner have been trying for a baby but so far have been unsuccessful. She is very tearful and mentions that her GP has recently started her on an anti-depressant.

Question 9:

A 30-year-old woman presents with a 3 month history of heavy periods associated with a cramping abdominal pain. She has regular cycles, bleeding 7/27 days. She has no inter-menstrual or post-coital bleeding. She changed her contraception 4 months ago.

For each of the following questions, choose the most likely cause of irregular menstrual bleeding. Each option may be used once, more than once or not at all.

Options:

1) Cervical cancer
2) Cervical polyp
3) Combined oral contraceptive pill
4) Ectropion
5) Endometrial cancer
6) Ovarian cancer
7) Ovarian cyst
8) Pelvic inflammatory disease
9) Physiological
10) Progesterone-only pill

Question 10:

A 35-year-old woman presents with a 3 month history of inter-menstrual bleeding and blood-stained, smelly vaginal discharge. She also describes post-coital bleeding. She has recently registered with a GP; before this, she has not been registered at any practice for some time. She has four children and is a heavy smoker. On examination there is an ulcer on the cervix.

Question 11:

A 32-year-old woman presents with a 4 month history of frequent periods. She is married. She is up to date with her smears and denies any dyspareunia, post-coital bleeding or discharge. She has recently changed contraceptive pill. Speculum and vaginal examination are normal.

Question 12:

A 52-year-old woman presents with irregular periods. She explains that her periods used to be 'regular as clockwork' but have become unpredictable over the past 6 months. She has missed a few periods and the bleeding has been heavier. She also reports dyspareunia. On examination, the vulva appears dry and sore and there is tenderness on vaginal examination.

For each of the following questions, choose the most likely cause of chronic pelvic pain. Each option may be used once, more than once or not at all.

Options:

1) Adenomyosis
2) Bladder stones
3) Endometriosis
4) Fibroids
5) Inflammatory bowel disease

6) Interstitial cystitis
7) Irritable bowel syndrome
8) Pelvic adhesions
9) Pelvic inflammatory disease
10) Psychological

Question 13:

A 25-year-old woman presents with a 12 month history of intermittent lower abdominal pain. The pain is cramping and associated with bloating and constipation. These episodes can happen at any time and last for a few days before improving. Her periods are regular (6/29) and have not changed over the past 12 months. She is tearful and complains of feeling tired all the time.

Question 14:

A 38-year-old woman presents with a 2 year history of chronic pelvic pain and heavy menstrual bleeding. Her pain is continuous but worsens during her period. She has a history of two caesarean sections and placenta accreta. On examination the uterus is bulky and tender. Transvaginal ultrasound shows a diffusely enlarged myometrium and elicits tenderness.

Question 15:

A 22-year-old woman presents with an 8 month history of bilateral pelvic pain. She also reports deep dyspareunia and inter-menstrual bleeding. She describes some yellowish vaginal discharge and has noticed that she tends to bleed after sex.

For each of the following questions, please pick the most likely cause of amenorrhoea. Each option may be used once, more than once or not at all.

Options:

1) Adrenal hyperplasia
2) Excessive exercise
3) Hyperthyroidism
4) Imperforate hymen
5) Polycystic ovary syndrome

6) Premature ovarian failure
7) Prolactinoma
8) Sheehan's syndrome
9) Stress
10) Turner's syndrome

Question 16:

A 21-year-old woman is concerned about her periods stopping recently. She has no medical conditions and a pregnancy test was negative. On further questioning, she mentions that she is training for a marathon and runs at least 6 miles each evening.

Question 17:

A 29-year-old woman presents with amenorrhoea. She has also noticed some acne on her face. Her body mass index is 35. You decide to do some blood tests and all of them come back normal, except testosterone and luteinizing hormone, which are both markedly raised.

Question 18:

A 16-year-old woman comes in with her mother. The mother is concerned that her daughter has not started her periods yet. You notice that the patient is very short and has some webbing of her neck. Blood tests show that her follicle-stimulating hormone and luteinizing hormone are elevated.

For each of the following questions, please pick the most likely cause of amenorrhoea. Each option may be used once, more than once or not at all.

Options:

1) Adrenal hyperplasia
2) Hyperandrogenism
3) Hyperinsulinaemia
4) Hypothyroidism
5) Imperforate hymen
6) Polycystic ovary syndrome
7) Premature ovarian failure
8) Prolactinoma
9) Sheehan's syndrome
10) Stress

Question 19:

A 25-year-old woman presents with amenorrhoea for the last 8 months. During this time she has noticed that she has been very tired. She mentions that she has joined a gym recently. Despite this, she has noticed some weight gain. Her skin has become very dry too. You notice that she has a slight neck swelling.

Question 20:

A 32-year-old chef is worried about her lack of periods. She already has three children and does not think she can handle another child. A pregnancy test is done and is negative. On further questioning, you discover that she has been finding it difficult to balance her working life with her family life.

Question 21:

A 30-year-old woman presents with a 9 month history of amenorrhoea. She also complains of headaches and changes to her vision. On examination, you find a bitemporal visual field defect. Blood tests show that her follicle-stimulating hormone and luteinizing hormone are low.

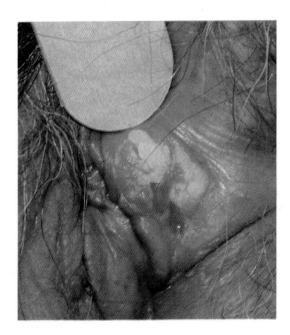

Fig. 22.1 **See Question 22.**

SBAs

Question 22:

What is the most likely cause of the lesion seen in Fig. 22.1?
1) Bartholinitis
2) Lichen planus
3) Lichen sclerosis
4) Lichen simplex
5) Vulval intra-epithelial neoplasia

Question 23:

A 30-year-old white woman presents with a 1 year history of heavy menstrual bleeding. The combined oral contraceptive pill and tranexamic acid prescribed by her GP have proven ineffective. On examination no pelvic mass is palpated; however, ultrasound scan confirms the presence of a large submucosal fibroid. What is the most appropriate management?
1) Gonadotrophin-releasing hormone agonists
2) Hysterectomy
3) Hysteroscopic removal
4) Myomectomy
5) Uterine artery embolization

Question 24:

Which of the following is **not** a risk factor for the development of endometrial cancer?
1) Combined oral contraceptive pill
2) Early menopause
3) Late menarche
4) Polycystic ovary syndrome
5) Tamoxifen

Question 25:

A 59-year-old woman presents with a long history of stress incontinence. Recently, this has worsened and she now also has symptoms of urgency and urge incontinence. She has two children, the first of whom was a ventouse delivery. On examination the vaginal cavity is normal with no evidence of major prolapse. Her body mass index is 30, but she is otherwise fit. What is the most likely diagnosis?
1) Cystourethrocele
2) Genuine stress incontinence
3) Mixed urinary incontinence
4) Overactive bladder
5) Urinary tract infection

Question 26:

A 58-year-old woman is currently under investigation for a long history of stress and urge incontinence. Mid-stream urine was negative for a urinary tract infection. Cystometry revealed urine flow on coughing in the absence of a detrusor contraction. She is normally fit and well but is a smoker. Her body mass index is 32. What is the most appropriate management?
1) Anti-muscarinic drugs, e.g. tolterodine
2) Bladder drill
3) Duloxetine
4) Supervised pelvic floor exercises
5) Tension-free vaginal tape

Question 27:

A 43-year-old woman presents with a 6 month history of heavy periods. When bleeding she uses tampons and pads, changing them hourly, and has occasional episodes of flooding. She complains of tiredness. Her periods are regular (5/30) and accompanied by some cramping pelvic pain. She denies inter-menstrual and post-coital bleeding. She was sterilized 4 years ago. Vaginal examination is normal. Which of the following is the most appropriate management of her heavy menstrual bleeding?

1) Endometrial biopsy
2) Gonadotrophin-releasing hormone analogue.
3) Hysterectomy
4) Intra-uterine system
5) Tranexamic acid

Question 28:

A 30-year-old nulliparous woman presents with a 3 year history of heavy periods and dysmenorrhoea. She and her partner are also concerned because she has not become pregnant in over 18 months of trying. Her GP has prescribed tranexamic acid and mefenamic acid to no effect. Pelvic examination is unremarkable. Her GP wonders whether she may have endometriosis. How would this be diagnosed?
1) Hysteroscopy
2) Laparoscopy
3) Pelvic ultrasound
4) Serum CA-125
5) Transvaginal ultrasound

Question 29:

A 39-year-old woman presents with post-coital bleeding. She has also noticed some spotting of blood between her periods, and complains of dyspareunia. She has undergone bimanual and speculum examination. Which of the following investigations is imperative?
1) Cervical cytology
2) Endometrial biopsy
3) Hysteroscopy
4) Pelvic ultrasound
5) Triple swabs

Question 30:

A 30-year-old nulliparous woman is referred to the early pregnancy assessment unit. She is 11 weeks pregnant. She has severe cramping pain in her lower abdomen and heavy vaginal bleeding. She has noticed some clots in the blood. On examination the uterus is just palpable abdominally. The cervical os is open. On transvaginal ultrasound the fetal heart beat can be seen. What is the most likely diagnosis?
1) Complete miscarriage
2) Incomplete miscarriage
3) Inevitable miscarriage
4) Missed miscarriage
5) Threatened miscarriage

Question 31:

An 85-year-old multiparous woman presents with a 12 month history of discomfort and feeling a lump 'down below'. She has tried to lose some weight and do pelvic floor exercises, but has not noticed any improvement in her symptoms. Vaginal examination identifies a second-degree uterine prolapse. She has a history of ischaemic heart disease and chronic obstructive pulmonary disease. What is the most appropriate management in this case?

1) Anterior repair
2) Hysterectomy
3) Pessary
4) Posterior repair
5) Sacrospinous colpopexy

Question 32:

A 53-year-old woman presents with menopausal symptoms. She has not had a period for 13 months. She complains of hot flushes, night sweats and dyspareunia. Her husband has noticed that she has become more irritable too. She was wondering whether there was anything she could take for these symptoms. Other than an appendectomy, she has no other past medical history. Which of the following would you recommend?

1) Bilateral salpingectomy
2) Hysterectomy
3) Oestrogen and progesterone (combined hormone replacement therapy)
4) Oestrogen-only hormone replacement therapy
5) Topical oestrogen

Answers

EMQs

Answer 1:

5) **Laparoscopy:** the likely diagnosis in this case is ectopic pregnancy, as all viable pregnancies should be visualized if the serum human chorionic gonadotrophin level is >1500 iu. Laparoscopy is required in order to investigate further and remove the ectopic from the tube. See Ectopic pregnancy in Chapter 16, Disorders of early pregnancy.

Answer 2:

6) **Laparotomy:** this patient is haemodynamically unstable; therefore, a laparotomy is urgently required. See Ectopic pregnancy in Chapter 16, Disorders of early pregnancy.

Answer 3:

7) **Methotrexate:** this is the most appropriate management in this case. The patient is suitable because she is haemodynamically stable and has a human chorionic gonadotrophin level <3000 iu. Laparoscopy would not be appropriate as she has only one fallopian tube and wishes to conserve her fertility. See Ectopic pregnancy in Chapter 16, Disorders of early pregnancy.

Answer 4:

9) **Transvaginal ultrasound:** in any woman presenting with post-menopausal bleeding it is essential to exclude endometrial carcinoma. Transvaginal ultrasound scan is the first-line investigation for endometrial carcinoma. If the endometrium is >5 mm thick a pipelle biopsy is taken, with/without hysteroscopy depending on the adequacy of the specimen. See Endometrial carcinoma in Chapter 14, Gynaecological malignancies.

Answer 5:

2) **Cervical smear:** any woman with post-coital bleeding should have abdominal pelvic examination and cervical smear to look for dyskaryosis. Triple swabs are also an appropriate initial investigation to exclude a sexually transmitted infection. See Cervical intra-epithelial neoplasia in Chapter 14, Gynaecological malignancies.

Answer 6:

1) **Abdominal/pelvic ultrasound:** ovarian cancer often presents in the late stages with non-specific abdominal symptoms. In a woman of this age an abdominal/pelvic ultrasound is indicated to exclude an ovarian mass. If an ovarian cancer is suspected the risk of malignancy index should be used to predict whether the mass is malignant. Ultrasound features, CA-125 and menopausal status are used to calculate the score. See Ovarian carcinoma in Chapter 14, Gynaecological malignancies.

Answer 7:

5) **Fibroids:** these are a common cause of heavy menstrual bleeding. This is a classic presentation of fibroids, which are more common in Afro-Caribbean women. An ovarian tumour may also present in its late stage as an abdominal mass. However, it is uncommon for ovarian tumours to cause menstrual irregularities. Ultrasound is the first-line investigation and will confirm the origin of the mass. See Fibroids in Chapter 13, Benign gynaecological disease.

Answer 8:

4) **Endometriosis:** this is the most likely diagnosis. The woman's age and the history of pain and infertility are typical of endometriosis. Pelvic inflammatory disease (PID) also causes deep dyspareunia and infertility. Although the symptoms of PID can be non-specific, it is more likely to cause inter-menstrual bleeding than heavy menstrual bleeding. Furthermore, there is no history of unusual vaginal discharge. This woman is also outside the typical 'high-risk' group of 15–24 years for PID. Endometriosis is the most likely diagnosis. See Endometriosis in Chapter 13, Benign gynaecological disease.

Answer 9:

7) **Intra-uterine coil device** (IUCD): this may cause heavier, longer and more painful periods in the first 3–6 months after insertion. Prescribing a non-steroidal anti-inflammatory drug or anti-fibrinolytic may reduce the bleeding, but if symptoms persist removal of the IUCD may be required. If appropriate, insertion of a Mirena® may be considered. There are no other symptoms, so the history is not suggestive of any underlying pelvic pathology. See Heavy menstrual bleeding in Chapter 12, Disorders of the menstrual cycle; Intra-uterine coil devices in Chapter 18, Contraception.

Answer 10:

1) **Cervical cancer:** this can be diagnosed in younger women. In the UK, the majority of cervical cancers are diagnosed by the screening programme. Symptoms are uncommon unless the cancer is advanced. The patient's increased parity and smoking status are risk factors for cervical cancer. An ectropion may present with inter-menstrual bleeding and discharge; however, on examination it is seen as a red ring on the ectocervix rather than an ulcer. Endometrial cancer is more common in post-menopausal women. See Cervical cancer in Chapter 14, Gynaecological malignancies.

Answer 11:

10) **Progesterone-only pill** (POP): erratic bleeding caused by the POP is the most likely diagnosis. Although pelvic inflammatory disease can cause irregular bleeding, the patient is not in a high-risk group and has no other suggestive symptoms, e.g. dyspareunia, vaginal discharge. Although an ectropion or polyp fit with the history, they would be seen on examination. See Irregular and inter-menstrual bleeding in Chapter 12, Disorders of the menstrual cycle; Hormonal contraception in Chapter 18, Contraception.

Answer 12:

9) **Physiological:** this woman is peri-menopausal. The first symptom of menopause is often irregular periods, which are the result of anovulatory cycles. Oestrogen deficiency causes vaginal atrophy, resulting in dryness and

dyspareunia. See Menopause in Chapter 11, Reproductive endocrinology; Irregular and inter-menstrual bleeding in Chapter 12, Disorders of the menstrual cycle.

Answer 13:

7) **Irritable bowel syndrome:** the lack of menstrual symptoms suggests that the origin of her pain is not gynaecological. Irritable bowel syndrome is the most likely diagnosis. It causes episodes of abdominal pain and cramping. This is usually associated with a change in bowel habit and lasts for a few days at a time. Inflammatory bowel disease would also cause chronic abdominal pain but is typically associated with diarrhoea and blood or mucus in the stool. See Dysmenorrhoea in Chapter 12, Disorders of the menstrual cycle.

Answer 14:

1) **Adenomyosis:** chronic pelvic pain associated with heavy menstrual bleeding (HMB) is suggestive of adenomyosis or endometriosis. Fibroids cause HMB but are rarely painful (the exceptions are during pregnancy or red degeneration). The most likely diagnosis in this woman is adenomyosis. Her obstetric history suggests she may have uterine damage, which is a risk factor for adenomyosis. The ultrasound result is consistent with a diagnosis of adenomyosis (note that there are no absolute diagnostic features for adenomyosis on ultrasound). Adenomyosis can be assessed with MRI and confirmed histologically after hysterectomy. See Adenomyosis in Chapter 13, Benign gynaecological disease.

Answer 15:

9) **Pelvic inflammatory disease** (PID): this is a classic history of PID, which typically presents in women under 24 years old. It is important to remember that PID can also be asymptomatic, particularly if *Chlamydia trachomatis* is the causative organism. See Irregular and inter-menstrual bleeding in Chapter 12, Disorders of the menstrual cycle; Pelvic inflammatory disease in Chapter 19, Genital tract infections.

Answer 16:

2) **Excessive exercise:** this is an example of hypogonadotrophic hypogonadism. Excessive exercise can switch off hypothalamic production of gonadotrophin-releasing hormone, leading to low gonadotrophin levels. This may be a protective measure to avoid pregnancy in an environment that the body perceives as inappropriate. Also, if the body mass index drops below 18 the periods may stop. See Amenorrhoea in Chapter 11, Reproductive endocrinology.

Answer 17:

5) **Polycystic ovary syndrome** (PCOS): this woman has features of PCOS. In addition to her amenorrhoea, she has both clinical (acne) and biochemical

Self-assessment

(raised testosterone) hirsutism and is also obese. See Polycystic ovary syndrome in Chapter 11, Reproductive endocrinology.

Answer 18:

10) **Turner's syndrome:** this can present soon after birth or around the time of delayed puberty. Short stature and neck webbing is typical. As the ovaries are unable to produce oestrogen, there is no negative feedback to limit follicle-stimulating hormone and luteinizing hormone secretion. See Amenorrhoea in Chapter 11, Reproductive endocrinology.

Answer 19:

4) **Hypothyroidism:** this woman is presenting with some hallmark features of hypothyroidism. Thyroid function tests would help to confirm the diagnosis. See Amenorrhoea in Chapter 11, Reproductive endocrinology.

Answer 20:

10) **Stress:** the most likely cause of this woman's amenorrhoea is stress, which causes hypogonadotrophic hypogonadism. See Amenorrhoea in Chapter 11, Reproductive endocrinology.

Answer 21:

8) **Prolactinoma:** this woman has a prolactinoma, which is a pituitary tumour that secretes prolactin. The tumour is pressing on the optic chiasm, which results in a characteristic bitemporal hemianopia. Prolactin inhibits the release of gonadotrophin-releasing hormone from the hypothalamus, resulting in low follicle-stimulating hormone and luteinizing hormone levels. It is worth noting that prolactinomas are more likely to be microprolactinomas (<10 mm) than macroprolactinomas (>10 mm), so in many cases there may not be any visual symptoms. See Amenorrhoea in Chapter 11, Reproductive endocrinology.

SBAs

Answer 22:

5) **Vulval intra-epithelial neoplasia** (VIN): Fig. 22.1 demonstrates eroded red areas and indurated pigmented lesions on the labia, which are typical characteristics of VIN. See Vulval intra-epithelial neoplasia in Chapter 14, Reproductive endocrinology.

Answer 23:

3) **Hysteroscopic removal:** depending on the size, this is the most appropriate management option for submucosal fibroids. Hysterectomy and uterine artery embolization are not recommended in women who may wish to conserve their

fertility. Gonadotrophin-releasing hormone agonists are usually limited to use in preparation for surgery. See Fibroids in Chapter 13, Benign gynaecological disease.

Answer 24:

1) **Combined oral contraceptive pill** (COCP): endometrial carcinoma results from the action of oestrogen on the uterus when unopposed by the protective effect of progesterone. The COCP and pregnancy have a protective effect on the endometrium whereas all the other factors listed above are risk factors. See Endometrial carcinoma in Chapter 14, Gynaecology malignancies.

Answer 25:

2) **Genuine stress incontinence** (GSI): although this patient has mixed symptoms the predominant feature is stress incontinence. Previous instrumental delivery and obesity are also risk factors for the development of GSI. Urinary tract infection should be excluded but it is unlikely given the long-standing nature of her symptoms. Cystometry is ultimately required to elucidate the cause. See Stress urinary incontinence in Chapter 15, Urogynaecology.

Answer 26:

4) **Supervised pelvic floor exercises:** genuine stress incontinence is the most likely cause of this woman's symptoms; therefore, anti-muscarinic drugs and a bladder drill would not be suitable. Pelvic floor exercises are the most appropriate initial management. Tension-free vaginal tape can be considered if this fails. Duloxetine may be offered as a second-line agent in women who do not wish to undergo surgery. The patient should also be counselled on lifestyle measures, e.g. weight loss. See Stress urinary incontinence in Chapter 15, Urogynaecology.

Answer 27:

4) **Intra-uterine system** (IUS): this woman has no signs or symptoms to indicate underlying pelvic pathology. She is therefore suitable for medical management. According to National Institute for Health and Clinical Excellence guidelines the first-line treatment should be the IUS, since she is not trying to conceive. In practice, many GPs and gynaecologists might try mefenamic acid, tranexamic acid or the combined oral contraceptive pill first. Hysterectomy might be indicated if medical management fails. Endometrial biopsy should always be considered for HMB. However, there are no indications for endometrial biopsy at this stage in this patient's management. See Heavy menstrual bleeding in Chapter 12, Disorders of the menstrual cycle.

Answer 28:

2) **Laparoscopy:** although a pelvic ultrasound would usually be done first, direct visualization of the pelvis by laparoscopy is the gold standard for diagnosis. Suspicious lesions are biopsied. Tubal patency can also be checked. See Endometriosis in Chapter 13, Benign gynaecological disease.

Answer 29:

1) **Cervical cytology:** these symptoms may be caused by cervical carcinoma. Although other aetiologies are possible, e.g. infection, ectropion and cervical polyp, cervical carcinoma should always be excluded in women with post-coital bleeding. Colposcopy may also be indicated, especially if a cervical lesion is seen on vaginal examination or the cytology result is abnormal. See Cervical cancer in Chapter 14, Gynaecological malignancies.

Answer 30:

3) **Inevitable miscarriage:** this woman is in the process of miscarriage. Although a fetal heart beat is seen the cervical os is open so miscarriage is inevitable. Threatened miscarriage presents with less pain and bleeding. Significantly, the cervical os will be closed so the pregnancy may remain viable. See Miscarriage in Chapter 16, Disorders of early pregnancy.

Answer 31:

3) **Pessary:** the definitive treatment of uterine prolapse is hysterectomy. However, this woman is unlikely to be medically fit for surgery. Trial of a ring pessary would be appropriate management in this case. See Uterovaginal prolapse in Chapter 15, Urogynaecology.

Answer 32:

3) **Oestrogen and progesterone:** oestrogen and progesterone would be the most appropriate form of hormone replacement therapy for this woman. She has some systemic symptoms (night sweats, mood swings), so topical oestrogen would not be suitable. There is no history of a hysterectomy so oestrogen must be given with progesterone. Remember that unopposed oestrogen can lead to endometrial hyperplasia/carcinoma. The first two options will not help with her symptoms. See Menopause in Chapter 11, Reproductive endocrinology.

Women's health

Questions

EMQs

For each clinical presentation what is the most appropriate diagnosis? Options may be used once, more than once or not at all.

Options:

1) Breast abscess
2) Breast cyst
3) Fat necrosis
4) Fibroadenoma
5) Invasive adenocarcinoma
6) Lymphoma
7) Mastitis
8) Nipple eczema
9) Paget's disease of the nipple
10) Sebaceous cyst

Question 1:

A 29-year-old woman presents with a painless lump in her right breast; on examination you note the mass is 3 cm in diameter, symmetrical and mobile.

Question 2:

A 72-year-old woman presents to her GP having recently noticed a change in the shape of her left breast. On examination you note dimpling of the skin in the lower quadrant of the breast and inversion of the nipple on the left.

Question 3:

A 33-year-old woman presents to the Accident and Emergency Department with an acutely painful right breast. She has been breast-feeding for 2 months. On examination her temperature is 38.5°C and the peri-areolar region is warm, swollen and tender.

SBAs

Question 4:

A 29-year-old woman is struggling to remember to take her combined oral contraceptive pill. She has come to seek an alternative form of contraception, but is reluctant to try a coil. She mentions that she has recently got engaged and expects to start a family in the next year. Which of the following forms of contraception would you recommend?
1) Contraceptive injection (e.g. Depo-Provera®)
2) Female sterilization
3) Intra-uterine system
4) Progesterone-only pill
5) Subdermal contraceptive implant (Nexplanon®)

Question 5:

A 24-year-old woman comes to your clinic and asks for some regular contraception. She is a non-smoker. She suffers from asthma and also has irregular periods, which can be quite heavy. Which of the following forms of contraception would you recommend?
1) Combined oral contraceptive pill
2) Contraceptive injection (Depo-Provera®)
3) Intra-uterine coil device
4) Intra-uterine system
5) Progesterone-only pill

Question 6:

A 45-year-old woman would like your advice on her contraceptive options. She has five children and is adamant that her family is complete. She has tried the progesterone-only pill in the past but is reluctant to go on any hormonal treatment again. She is a smoker. Which of the following forms of contraception would you recommend?
1) Combined oral contraceptive pill
2) Contraceptive injection (Depo-Provera®)
3) Intra-uterine coil device
4) Intra-uterine system
5) Subdermal contraceptive implant (Nexplanon®)

Question 7:

A 20-year-old woman presents with vaginal discharge. There is no smell but she describes it as looking like 'thick cream'. There is also an associated itch. What is the most likely diagnosis?

1) Bacterial vaginosis
2) Candidiasis
3) Ectropion
4) Foreign body
5) Trichomoniasis

Question 8:

A 23-year-old woman presents with vaginal discharge. She also complains of some pelvic pain. On further questioning, she admits to having unprotected sex in the last few months with multiple partners. What is the most likely diagnosis?
1) Bacterial vaginosis
2) Chlamydia
3) Ectropion
4) Foreign body
5) Human immunodeficiency virus

Question 9:

What does Fig. 23.1 show?

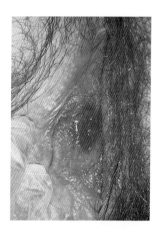

Fig. 23.1 See Question 9.

1) Bacterial vaginosis
2) Candidiasis
3) Genital warts
4) Gonorrhoea
5) Primary syphilis

Question 10:

You suspect that your 26-year-old female patient has gonorrhoea. Which of the following would help to confirm your diagnosis?

1) Endocervical swab
2) Full blood count
3) High vaginal swab
4) Urine dipstick
5) Venereal Disease Research Laboratory test

Question 11:

A 32-year-old woman presents with a grey–white vaginal discharge. She mentions that the discharge smells like fish. You perform a 'whiff' test, which is positive. What is the most likely diagnosis?

1) Bacterial vaginosis
2) Ectropion
3) Foreign body
4) Gonorrhoea
5) Trichomoniasis

Question 12:

A 63-year-old woman presents to her GP with an itchy red nipple on the left breast, and requests some cream for this. On examination you note that the eczematous rash is unilateral and involves both the areola and nipple. What is the most likely diagnosis?

1) Atopic dermatitis
2) Nipple eczema
3) Paget's disease of the nipple
4) Psoriasis
5) Scabies

Question 13:

A 55-year-old woman presents with a hard irregular lump in the upper outer quadrant of her right breast. You note that she attended the Accident and Emergency Department 1 month previously with whiplash after a road traffic accident. On examination the mass is mobile and firm. What is the most likely diagnosis?

1) Breast abscess
2) Breast cyst
3) Fat necrosis
4) Fibrous nodularity
5) Invasive adenocarcinoma

Question 14:

A 47-year-old woman presents with a lump in the lower outer quadrant of her left breast. On examination the lump is smooth; mammography shows a radiolucent ring surrounding the mass. What is the most likely diagnosis?
1) Breast abscess
2) Breast cyst
3) Fat necrosis
4) Invasive adenocarcinoma
5) Paget's disease of the nipple

Answers

EMQs

Answer 1:

4) **Fibroadenoma:** these are the most common breast tumour in women of child-bearing age. They are hormone responsive and may increase in size cyclically or during pregnancy. They are commonly well defined with a symmetrical border and are mobile on palpation. Diagnosis is usually clinical but a fibroadenoma of >4 cm in diameter would warrant biopsy. See Fibroadenoma (Breast mouse) in Chapter 20, Diseases of the breast and their assessment and treatment.

Answer 2:

5) **Invasive adenocarcinoma:** the patient's age, skin dimpling and nipple inversion suggest locally advanced breast cancer, of which adenocarcinoma is the most common histological type. See Breast cancer in Chapter 20, Diseases of the breast and their assessment and treatment.

Answer 3:

1) **Breast abscess:** this patient's temperature and acutely swollen tender breast mass are suggestive of a breast abscess. Her recent history of breast-feeding increases this risk as bacteria are introduced into the breast and milk glands become blocked. See Mastitis and breast abscess in Chapter 20, Diseases of the breast and their assessment and treatment.

SBAs

Answer 4:

5) **Subdermal contraceptive implant:** remember that patient choice should always be taken into account when giving contraceptive advice. Since this

woman is reluctant to try a coil, the intra system is ruled out. Sterilization is not suitable for obvious reasons. It would also be unwise to recommend the progesterone-only pill when she is already having trouble remembering to take the combined oral contraceptive pill. Only two options are left: subdermal contraceptive implant or contraceptive injection. The fact that she wants to start a family soon means that the subdermal contraceptive implant device would be the more appropriate of the two. There is a rapid return to fertility after removal of the device, but it can take up to 2 years for fertility to return after stopping the injections. See Subdermal contraceptive implant (Nexplanon®) in Chapter 18, Contraception.

Answer 5:

1) **Combined oral contraceptive pill** (COCP): this woman would be suitable for trial of the COCP as she is a non-smoker and there is no history of venous thrombosis or migraines. The COCP will also help to regulate her periods and reduce her menorrhagia. The progesterone-only options (progesterone-only pill, intra-uterine system and contraceptive injection) may cause more erratic bleeding and the intra-uterine coil device may lead to longer and more painful periods. See Combined oral contraceptive pill in Chapter 18, Contraception.

Answer 6:

3) **Intra-uterine coil device** (IUCD): this is the only non-hormonal form of contraception out of the options available. Women over the age of 40 may retain the IUCD until they no longer need contraception. These patients can wait until they have undergone the menopause before having the device removed. If male or female sterilization had been options, both would have been worth consideration in this scenario. See Intra-uterine coil devices in Chapter 18, Contraception.

Answer 7:

2) **Candidiasis:** this history is typical of candidiasis, which is also known as thrush. It is usually caused by infection with *Candida albicans*. The classic description of the discharge is 'cottage cheese'. See Candidiasis (Thrush) in Chapter 19, Genital tract infections.

Answer 8:

2) **Chlamydia**: the symptoms and signs that this patient presents with, along with her history of unprotected sex, point towards a diagnosis of a sexually transmitted infection. While it is possible that she may have human immunodeficiency virus, it is unlikely to present in this way. Chlamydia commonly presents asymptomatically, but it is important to remember that it can present with vaginal discharge and pelvic pain. See Chlamydia in Chapter 19, Genital tract infections.

Answer 9:

3) **Genital warts:** Fig. 23.1 shows multiple lesions that range from being flat to papilliform. Genital warts can present like this and the lumps are usually painless. It can be easily treated with topical podophyllin or cryotherapy. It cannot be primary syphilis as that usually presents with a solitary ulcer known as a chancre. See Genital warts (Condylomata accuminata) in Chapter 19, Genital tract infections.

Answer 10:

1) **Endocervical swab:** to confirm a diagnosis of gonorrhoea, endocervical specimens are required for either microscopy or culture, so you would need to do an endocervical swab. A urine dipstick and a full blood count may show signs of infection but would not help with confirming your diagnosis of gonorrhoea. A Venereal Disease Research Laboratory test is a serological test specifically used for diagnosing syphilis, so would not help in this case either. See Gonorrhoea in Chapter 19, Genital tract infections.

Answer 11:

1) **Bacterial vaginosis:** these features are typical of bacterial vaginosis. You would also see 'clue cells' on microscopy. See Bacterial vaginosis in Chapter 19, Genital tract infections.

Answer 12:

3) **Paget's disease of the nipple:** the presentation of unilateral eczematous changes of the nipple with both areola and nipple involvement is highly suggestive of Paget's disease, which is commonly associated with an underlying ductal carcinoma of the breast. Nipple eczema is commonly bilateral and involves just the areola and not the nipple. See Paget's disease of the nipple in Chapter 20, Diseases of the breast and their assessment and treatment.

Answer 13:

3) **Fat necrosis:** this commonly follows trauma or surgery to the breast. The lump is usually hard and irregular and may be tethered to the skin. Overlying bruising or shrinkage of the mass is suggestive of fat necrosis, but biopsy may be required to exclude carcinoma. This will show the presence of inflammatory cells. See Fat necrosis in Chapter 20, Diseases of the breast and their assessment and treatment.

Answer 14:

2) **Breast cyst:** these are common in the peri-menopausal period and are smooth and fluctuant on examination. Mammography will show the typical halo sign: a radiolucent ring surrounding the cyst. See Breast cysts in Chapter 20, Diseases of the breast and their assessment and treatment.

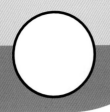

Bibliography

1993 Revised Classification System for HIV Infection and Expanded Surveillance Case Definition for AIDS Among Adolescents and Adults: http://www.cdc.gov/mmwr/preview/mmwrhtml/00018871.htm Accessed 18/8/2010

Adjuvant online. http://www.adjuvantonline.com/index.jsp

Amniocentisis – complications. http://www.nhs.uk/Conditions/Amniocentesis/Pages/Complications.aspx Accessed April 2012.

Baker P. *Obstetrics by Ten Teachers*. 18th edition. London: Hodder Arnold, 2006

Baker P. Kenny L. *Obstetrics by Ten Teachers*. 19th edition. London: Hodder Arnold, 2011.

Birth Control Trust. Abortion Provision in Britain – How services are provided and how they could be improved. London: Birth Control Trust; 1997.

Cancer Research UK. Breast cancer statistics. http://info.cancerresearchuk.org/cancerstats/types/breast

Chorionic villus sampling and amniocentesis: information for you. http://www.rcog.org.uk/womens-health/clinical-guidance/chorionic-villus-sampling-cvs-what-you-need-know. Accessed April 2012

Clinical Knowledge Summaries. Management of stress urinary incontinence symptoms. Available at: http://www.cks.nhs.uk/incontinence_urinary_in_women/management/detailed_answers/secondary_care_treatments_for_urgency_incontinence#-368673.

Clinical Knowledge Summaries. Endometriosis. Available at http://www.cks.nhs.uk/endometriosis. Accessed May 2011

Clinical Knowledge Summaries. Miscarriage. Available at http://www.cks.nhs.uk/miscarriage.

Collier J., Longmore M., Turmezei T., Mafi A. Gynaecology. In *Oxford Handbook of Clinical Specialities*. Eighth edition. Oxford: Oxford University Press, 2009.

Collier J. Longmore M. Turmezei T. Mafi A. Obsetrics. In *Oxford Handbook of Clinical Specialities*. Eighth edition. Oxford: Oxford University Press, 2009.

Government Statistical Service. NHS Maternity Statistics, England: 2002–03. March 2004. Available at: http://www.dh.gov.uk/prod_consum_dh/groups/dh_digitalassets/@dh/@en/documents/digitalasset/dh_4080823.pdf

Hollingworth T. Lichen planus. Independent nurse. Available at: http://www.independentnurse.co.uk/cgibin/go.pl/library/articlehtml.cgi?uid=83330;type=Clinical

Hollingworth T. Vulval diseases – lichen sclerosus. Indpendent Nurse. Available at http://www.independentnurse.co.uk/cgibin/go.pl/library/articlehtml.cgi?uid=82775;type=Clinical

Hollingworth, T. Lichen simplex chonicus. Independent Nurse. Available at: http://www.independentnurse.co.uk/cgibin/go.pl/library/articlehtml.cgi?uid=84069;type=Clinical

Impey L. *Obstetrics & Gynaecology*. Second Edition. Oxford: Wiley-Blackwell, 2004.

Impey L. and Child T. *Obstetrics & Gynaecology*. 3rd edn. UK: Wiley-Blackwell, 2008.

Kumar P and Clark M (eds.). *Clinical Medicine*. 6th edn. Edinburgh: Elsevier. Saunders.

MedlinePlus [Internet]. Bethesda (MD): National Library of Medicine (US); [updated 21/11/2010]. Miscarriage. Accessed August 2011. Available from: http://www.nlm.nih.gov/medlineplus/ency/article/001488.htm.

MeReC (2003) Tackling premenstrual syndrome. 'MeReC Bulletin' 13(3), 9–12. Available at http://www.npc.nhs.uk/merec/other_non_clinical/resources/merec_bulletin_vol13_no3.pdf. Accessed May 2011.

Monga A. *Gynaecology by Ten Teachers.* 18th edition. London: Hodder Arnold, 2006

Monga A. and Dobbs S. *Gynaecology by Ten Teachers.* 19th edition. London: Hodder Arnold, 2011.

National Institute for Health and Clinical Excellence. Familial Breast Cancer. NICE guideline 41. London UK, NICE 2006. Available at: http://www.nice.org.uk/nicemedia/pdf/CG41NICEguidance/pdf.

NHS CRD (1995) Management of menorrhagia. Effective Health Care 1(9), 1–15. Available at: http://www.york.ac.uk/inst/crd/EHC/ehc19.pdf. Accessed April 2011

Clinical Knowledge Summaries. Dysmennorhoea. http://www.cks.nhs.uk/dysmenorrhoea#-449687. Accessed May 2011.

NHS Fetal Anomaly Screening Programme. Online CEMT21 Training Resource. Available at: http://fetalanomaly.screening.nhs.uk/CEMT21/. Accessed March 2011.

Proctor M. and Farquhar C. Diagnosis and management of dysmenorrhoea. *British Medical Journal.* 2006; 332(7550), 1134–1138

Roberts C L, Bell J C, Ford J B *et al.* The accuracy of reporting of the hypertensive disorders of pregnancy in population health data. *Hypertension in Pregnancy.* 2008; 27(3): 285–97.

Sarris I., Bewley S., Agnihotri S. *Training in Obstetrics and Gynaecology the essential curriculum.* Oxford: Oxford University Press, 2009.

Society of Obstetricians and Gynaecologists of Canada. Consensus Guidelines for the Management of Chronic Pelvic Pain. Available at http://www.sogc.org/guidelines/public/164e-cpg1-august2005.pdf.

Statutory Instrument 2002 No. 887. The Abortion (Amendment) (England) Regulations 2002. London: HMSO; 2002 [http://www.hmso.gov.uk/si/si2002/20020887.htm].

Vessey MP., Villard-Mackintosh L., McPherson K. *et al.* The epidemiology of hysterectomy: findings in a large cohort study. *British Journal of Obstetrics & Gynaecology.* 1992; 99(5), 402–407.

Wittekind, C., Greene, F.L., Hutter, R.V.P., Klimpfinger, M., and Sobin, L.H. (2004). Breast Tumours. In *TNM Atlas Illustrated Guide to the TNM/pTNM Classification of Malignant tumours.* C. Wittekind, F.L. Greene, R.V.P. Hutter, M. Klimpfinger, and L.H. Sobin, (eds). New York: Springer, 2004, pp. 207–224.

Index

Note: Page numbers with brackets e.g. 286(288-9), are to questions with the answer indicated in brackets. On some occasions, the indexed topic does not appear in the question itself but is listed in the EMQ options on a preceding page.